NEW DIRECTIONS IN HEALTH PSYCHOLOGY ASSESSMENT

Series in Applied Psychology: Social Issues and Questions

Stevan Hobfoll, *Editor-in-Chief*

Schroeder New Directions in Health Psychology Assessment
Stephens, Crowther, Hobfoll, Tennenbaum Stress and Coping in Later-Life Families

IN PREPARATION

Crowther, Hobfoll, Stephens, Tennenbaum Bulimia Nervosa: The Individual and Familial Context

NEW DIRECTIONS IN HEALTH PSYCHOLOGY ASSESSMENT

Edited by

Harold E. Schroeder, Ph.D.

Kent State University, Ohio

HEMISPHERE PUBLISHING CORPORATION

A member of the Taylor & Francis Group

New York Washington Philadelphia London

NEW DIRECTIONS IN HEALTH PSYCHOLOGY ASSESSMENT

1 2 3 4 5 6 7 8 9 0 B R B R 9 8 7 6 5 4 3 2 1 0

This book was set in Times Roman by Hemisphere Publishing Corporation. The editors were Andrew N. Bartlett and Susan Bedford; the designer was Debra Eubanks Riffe; the production supervisor was Peggy M. Rote; and the typesetters were Linda Andros and Wayne Hutchins.
Cover design by Debra Eubanks Riffe.
Printing and binding by Braun Brumfield, Inc.

A CIP catalog record for this book is available from the British Library.

Library of Congress Cataloging-in-Publication Data

New directions in health psychology assessment / edited by Harold E. Schroeder.
p. cm. — (Series in applied psychology)
Based on a conference held at Kent State University in 1987; sponsored by the Applied Psychology Center of the Dept. of Psychology, Kent State University.
Includes bibliographical references.
Includes index.

1. Health risk assessment—Philosophy—Congresses. 2. Health status indicators—Evaluation—Congresses. I. Schroeder, Harold E. II. Kent State University, Applied Psychology Center. III. Series: Series in applied psychology (New York, N.Y.)
[DNLM: 1. Health Policy—United States—congresses. 2. Mental Health—United States—congresses. 3. Outcome and Process Assessment (Health Care)—methods—congresses. 4. Outcome and Process Assessment (Health Care)—trends—congresses. W 84 AA1 N45 1987]
RA427.3.N48 1991
362.1′042—dc20
DNLM/DLC
for Library of Congress

ISBN 0-89116-925-3
ISSN 1048-8146

Contents

Contributors

GARY W. EVANS, Program in Social Ecology, University of California at Irvine, Irvine, CA 92717

LEONARD A. JASON, Department of Psychology, DePaul University, Chicago, IL 60604

ROBERT M. KAPLAN, Division of Health Care Sciences, M-022, Department of Community and Family Medicine, University of California at San Diego, La Jolla, CA 92093

PAUL KAROLY, Department of Psychology, Arizona State University, Tempe, AZ 85287-1104

STANISLAV V. KASL, Department of Epidemiology and Public Health, Yale University School of Medicine, New Haven, CT 06510

WENDY KLIEWER, Program in Social Ecology, University of California at Irvine, Irvine, CA 92717

JANAEA MARTIN, Program in Social Ecology, University of California at Irvine, Irvine, CA 92717

DAVID H. OLSON, Family Social Science Department, University of Minnesota, St. Paul, MN 55108

JEAN E. RHODES, Department of Psychology, University of Illinois at Urbana-Champaign, Champaign, IL 61820

KENNETH L. STEWART, Child Development and Family Studies, North Dakota State University, Fargo, ND 58102

Preface

The area of health assessment initially did not appear to pose particular problems for health psychologists. Certain risk factors involving lifestyle behaviors or personality variables seemed obvious targets for intervention. Standard methods of behavior change seemed to be fairly effective initially in individual cases. When it later became apparent that some of these behaviors were resistant to change and that improvement in national health status was a complicated goal, new issues in assessment began to arise.

The targets of intervention are no longer obvious. As we look at various social systems such as the family or work, complex factors interact to produce health outcomes. Communities differ in their health needs, and it is not obvious how to identify them. Although most people would agree that our health may be affected by our physical environments, it is not clear which dimensions of the environments may be important at various ages. Individuals make many health decisions, but the bases for those decisions are difficult to assess. Health outcomes themselves are difficult to evaluate when the costs and benefits of various alternatives are considered.

Such issues became apparent at a conference on health assessment at Kent State University in 1987. The conference was held by the Applied Psychology Center of the Department of Psychology to examine the state of the art of measuring factors important to health. The focus was not on a survey of extant methods of assessing, say, quality of life but on the limitations of current methods and proposals for the future. The present volume is an outgrowth of that conference.

In the first chapter, Robert Kaplan proposes a model that can be used to quantify the health effects of various alternatives in health care. The model integrates point-in-time estimates of function, transitions among function levels over time, utilities for health states, and mortality outcomes. A particular value of the model is its integration of different components of health within a single unit. This General Health Policy model can be used to compare the values of very different alternatives in health care.

Stanislav Kasl describes the implications of a focus on specific physical health outcomes instead of our traditional focus on illness behaviors in the work environment. With the former, research must not only include biological parameters but also measure the work environment separately from perceptions and reactions to it. The field of occupational epidemiology is reviewed from this perspective to identify pathogenic work dimensions that affect specific biological variables rather than behaviors such as absenteeism or medical care-seeking.

While there is considerable evidence of a relationship between physical environmental conditions and health for adults, considerably less attention has been given to child health outcomes. The health implications of child–environment transactions are reviewed by Gary Evans, Wendy Kliewer, and Janaea Martin. Highlighted in this review are ambient features of the physical environment; contextual features of school, the home, and outdoor environments such as playgrounds; and the factors that provide resilience to adverse environmental conditions.

Drawing on a family systems paradigm, David Olson and Kenneth Stewart review the impact of the family on health, health maintenance, and health behavior change. They also propose a Multisystem Assessment of Stress and Health (MASH) model for assessing stress, coping resources, and adaptation at four system levels: individual, family, marital, and work.

Challenging the assumptions and techniques of traditional assessment, Jean Rhodes and Leonard Jason discuss the assessment of community health needs from an ecological and collaborative framework. Following a review of the advantages and disadvantages of traditional methods, they suggest new methods that emphasize the use of community values, empowerment, and collaboration in the evaluation of community-based health promotion programs.

Finally, Paul Karoly proposes a goal-directed model for health behaviors. He suggests that a goal systems analysis can identify the functional, structural, and ecological attributes of goals that characterize a self-regulating system. A method of measuring goal systems is included.

This volume is intended primarily for students and researchers in the field of health psychology. It is not intended to be a comprehensive survey but rather an in-depth analysis of health assessment in areas where new directions are emerging. The present authors have outlined what these new directions are and suggested how they may be pursued.

I would like to express specific thanks to the Applied Psychology Center at Kent State. It was through the support of the center that this volume was made possible.

Harold E. Schroeder

1

ASSESSMENT OF QUALITY OF LIFE FOR SETTING PRIORITIES IN HEALTH POLICY

Robert M. Kaplan

University of California, San Diego

INTRODUCTION

Utility is a condition or quality of usefulness. High-utility items are the most useful, and those with lower utility are less useful. States of being are also associated with utilities. Health is often identified as the highest utility asset. When Rokeach (1973) asked subjects to prioritize their values, he found no variability for the rank of health. It was always ranked first and, for this reason, was eventually removed from the Rokeach Value Scale. This chapter defines health and offers a quantitative expression of health status.

Because health is so highly valued, people will spend their energy and assets attempting to achieve it. In 1988, Americans spent $544 billion on health care services and a much larger amount on other products and services related to health. Although there is tremendous incentive to promote products and services as health-enhancing, we typically are left with little information about the extent to which health outcome is affected by these investments. Thus, another purpose of this chapter is to explore changes in a quantitative expression of health in relation to investments. First, let us consider variations in the use of expensive health care services across cultures and within the United States.

This work was supported, in part, by Grants RO1 HL34732 and AR 33489 from the National Institutes of Health. In addition, the work was completed while the author was supported, in part, by the California Policy Seminar. This chapter overlaps, in part, with previously published papers (Kaplan, 1989; Kaplan & Anderson, 1988a).

Small Area Variation Studies

It is typically assumed that the amount of health service consumed is a reflection of the need for the service. Thus, it would be expected that in demographically equivalent communities, the use of specific health care services would be approximately equal. However, Wennberg, Freeman, and Culp (1987) have shown that this is not the case. Within New England communities with demographically equivalent populations, the variation in the use of some services is substantial. For example, women in some communities are 9 times more likely to have a hysterectomy than are women with their same characteristics in a bordering community. Men with the same symptoms are 13 times more likely to have prostate operations in some communities than in others (Roos, 1984; Wennberg, 1990).

Is More Better?

One of the basic objectives in the area of health care is to deliver service. Indeed, many policy options are justified because they provide more services. We assume that expenditure is equivalent to accomplishment. The more money allocated to a program, the better the expected outcomes. It is often assumed that the states or countries that are achieving the best health outcomes are those spending the most money. Thus, it might be argued, Americans should have the world's best health profile because they spend the most per capita on health care.

Recently, substantial evidence has emerged suggesting that many unnecessary services are delivered by our health care system. Consider coronary artery bypass surgery. In 1979, the United States Congress Office of Technology Assessment reported that in France there are 19 such operations per million members of the population. In Austria, there are 150 such operations per million in the population. In the United States, there are nearly 800 of these operations per million (Rimm, 1985). Approximately 200,000 bypass procedures were performed in the United States in 1985—nearly twice as many as had been performed in 1980 (National Center for Health Statistics, 1986). There are also large differences in the use of other expensive interventions. For example, the number of people with end-stage renal disease is believed to be approximately equal in Western countries. Yet in the United Kingdom, less than 1 case per 1,000 was on renal dialysis, in comparison with 39 cases per 1,000 in the United States (Schroeder, 1987). As argued by a variety of analysts, there is no evidence that these regional variations in use of procedures have substantial effects on health outcomes. They do have systematic effects upon health care costs.

Policy analysts are faced with difficult choices because they hope to maximize health outcomes while maintaining control over costs. Western countries differ in the rate at which health care costs have escalated. The United States now spends nearly 11% of its gross national product (GNP) on health care, while other countries with high technology medicine, such as Japan, spend only about 8%, and Great Britain spends about 6%. It is not clear that escalating expenditure has been associated with equal returns in health status. Among countries reporting data to the Organization for Economic Cooperation and Development, the shortest life expectancies for men are in Ireland and the longest are in Greece. Among the reporting nations, Greece paradoxically spends the smallest percentage of its GNP on health care, while Ireland spends the most. In fact, there is a rough negative relationship among the reporting nations between expenditures and life expectancy (Sick Health Services, 1988). Studies (reviewed by Voulgaropolous, Schneiderman, & Kaplan, 1989) have shown that many widely used and expensive procedures have essentially no health benefit.

In order to gain a better understanding of the alternatives in health care, we have proposed a General Health Policy Model that attempts to provide a comprehensive expression of the costs, risks, and benefits of competing alternatives in health care. Some of these choices are difficult without a model because comparing programs might be considered analogous to comparing apples to oranges.

Apples Versus Oranges

There are many alternative ways to spend money on health care. These range from complex, high technology interventions such as liver transplantation to rehabilitation to primary prevention. Comparing these alternatives might be analogous to comparing apples to oranges. Further complicating the comparison is the fact that the benefits of each intervention are measured in quite different units. Liver transplantation might be evaluated in terms of extended life expectancy. The successful procedure might be one in which the patient survives for one year. These procedures might require large expenditures for a single patient. The same amount of money might be spent to provide a different smaller benefit for a large number of people. Recently, for example, the state of Oregon was faced with a complex dilemma. They had a limited number of health care dollars and had to choose between high technology transplantation surgery and other alternatives, including prenatal care. Each liver transplant, for example, costs about $325,000. After deliberation, Oregon administrators decided to rank funding of prenatal care higher than some organ transplantation programs. Many people argued that this was a foolish decision. Yet, the systematic comparison between the benefits was not possible because the outcomes of the services were measured in quite different units. In the next sections, I will discuss models for thinking about these comparison problems. Ultimately, I will suggest that there are methods for quantifying health benefits and that the use of these models may serve to challenge many of our assumptions about health care. One of these assumptions is that we benefit from greater expenditures in health care.

Public policy makers are faced with complex decisions that often involve comparisons between very different alternatives. When these alternatives are measured or described using different scales, decisions can be difficult, if not impossible. Often, the confused decision-maker gives in to the most emotional appeal. In this chapter, I argue that general measurement models, based on behavioral measurement, can provide important new insights for policy makers. These models depend on general conceptualizations of the expected benefits or consequences of health care decisions. We have developed a General Health Policy Model (Kaplan & Anderson, 1988a) that quantitatively expresses the ultimate objectives of health care: to extend life expectancy and improve quality of life.

MEASUREMENT OF HEALTH STATUS

The conceptualization and measurement of health status has interested scholars for many decades. Following the Eisenhower administration, a President's Commission on National Goals identified health status measurement as an important objective. Shortly after, John Kenneth Galbraith, in *The Affluent Society* (1958), described the need to measure the effect of the health care system on quality of life. Recent years have seen many attempts to define and measure health state (Bergner, 1985; Walker & Rosser, 1988; Wenger, Mattson, Furberg, & Elinson, 1984). Before considering any specific approach, it is worth noting that traditional indictors of health have well identified problems.

Mortality

Mortality remains the major outcome measure in most epidemiologic studies and clinical trials. Typically, mortality is expressed as a unit of time. For mortality data to be meaningful, they must be expressed as a rate, that is, the proportion of deaths from a particular cause occurring in some defined time interval (usually a year). Mortality rates are often age-adjusted. Case fatality rates express the proportion of persons who died of a particular disease divided by the total number with the disease (including those who die and those who live). Reporting mortality rates has its advantages. They are "hard" data, despite some misclassification bias (National Institutes of Health, 1979) and the meaning of the outcome is not difficult to comprehend. Despite their many advantages, mortality outcomes have some obvious limitations. Mortality rates consider only the dead and ignore the living. Many important treatments or programs might have little or no impact on mortality rates, and some important illnesses (e.g., arthritis) have relatively little impact upon mortality.

Morbidity

The most common approach to health status assessment is to measure morbidity in terms of function or role performance. For example, morbidity estimates often include work days missed or bed disability days. Many different approaches to health status assessment using morbidity indicators have been introduced. These include, for example, the Sickness Impact Profile (Bergner, Bobbitt, Carter, & Gilson, 1981), which represents the effect of disease or disability upon a variety of categories of behavioral function; and the RAND Health Status Measures, which have separate categories for the effects of disease or health states upon physical function, social function, and mental function. These measures do not integrate morbidity and mortality, although as each birth cohort ages, mortality cases accrue.

Death is a health outcome, and it is important that this outcome be included in any expression of health status. For example, suppose we were evaluating the effect of Program A, integrated support and treatment, against that of Program B, no support or treatment, for randomly assigned groups of very ill, elderly, nursing home residents. Let us suppose that Program A maintained patients at a very low level of function throughout the year, but that in the comparison group (Program B), the sickest 10% died. Looking just at the living in the follow-up, one finds Program B patients to be healthier, since the sickest had been removed by death. By this standard, the program of no supportive treatment might be put forth as the better alternative. With a measure that combined morbidity and mortality the outcome would be very different, because mortality effects would reduce the overall health of Program B to a very low level.

Health-Related Quality of Life

The objectives of health care are two-fold. First, health care and health policy should increase life expectancy. Second, the health care system should improve the quality of life during the years that people are alive. It is instructive to consider various measures in health care in light of these two objectives. Traditional biomedical indictors and diagnoses are important to us because they may be related to mortality or to quality of life. We prefer the term *health-related quality of life* to refer to the impact of health conditions on function. Thus, health-related quality of life may be independent of quality of life relevant to work setting, housing, air pollution, or similar factors (Rice, 1984).

Numerous quality of life measurement systems have evolved during the last 20 years. These systems are based primarily on two different conceptual approaches. The first approach grows out of the tradition of health status measurement. In the late 1960s and early 1970s, the National Center for Health Services Research funded several major projects to develop general measures of health status. Those projects resulted in the Sickness Impact Profile (SIP) (Bergner, Bobbitt, Carter, & Gilson, 1981), the Quality of Well-being Scale (Kaplan & Bush, 1982), and the General Health Rating Index. The latter measure, originally developed at Southern Illinois University, was adapted by the RAND Corporation under ASPE grants and has become known as the RAND Health Status Measure (Stewart, Ware, Brook, & Davies-Avery, 1978). These efforts usually involved extensive multidisciplinary collaboration between behavioral scientists and physicians and, perhaps not surprisingly, most are focused on the impact of disease and disability on function and observable behaviors, such as performance of social role, ability to get around the community, and physical functioning. Some systems include separate components for the measurement of social and mental health. All were guided by the World Health Organization's (WHO) definition of health status: "Health is a complete state of physical, mental, and social well-being and not merely absence of disease" (World Health Organization, 1948).

The second conceptual approach is based upon quality of life as something independent of health status. Some investigators now use traditional psychological measures and call them "quality of life" outcomes. For instance, Follick, Gorkin, Smith, Capone, and Stabein (1988) suggest that quality of life represents psychological status in addition to symptoms and mortality. In fact, most investigators believe that symptoms and mortality do represent quality of life (Bush, 1984). Croog et al. (1986) used a wide variety of outcome measures and collectively referred to them as "quality of life." These measures included the patients' subjective evaluation of well-being, physical symptoms, sexual function, work performance and satisfaction, emotional status, cognitive function, social participation, and life satisfaction. Other investigators, including Hunt and colleagues (Hunt & McEwen, 1983) regard quality of life as subjective appraisals of life satisfaction. In summary, a wide variety of different dimensions have all been described as "quality of life." Although agreement is lacking on which dimensions should be considered the standard for assessing quality of life in research studies, recurrent themes in the methodological literature can assist in the evaluation of existing instruments.

Unidimensional Versus Multidimensional Constructs

Although all experts agree that quality of life is a multidimensional construct, they debate whether outcome measures must necessarily represent this multidimensional structure. Quality of life assessment can take essentially one of two major approaches: a psychometric approach or a decision theory approach. The psychometric or profile approach attempts to provide separate measures for the many different dimensions of quality of life. Perhaps the best known example of the psychometric tradition is the SIP, which is a 136-item measure that yields

12 different scores. The scores are displayed as a profile similar to a Minnesota Mutliphasic Personality Inventory (MMPI).

The decision theory approach attempts to weight the different dimensions of health to gain a single unitary expression of health status. Supporters of this approach argue that psychometric approaches fail to consider that different health problems are not of equal concern: one hundred runny noses are not the same as 100 severe abdominal pains (Bush, 1984). Not uncommonly, experimental trials using the psychometric approach will find that some aspects of quality of life improve while others get worse. For example, a medication might reduce high blood pressure but also be associated with headaches and impotence. The decision theory approach attempts to place an overall value on health status by weighting the different dimensions and combining them into an aggregate quality score on the grounds that the "quality" notion is the subjective evaluation of observable or objective health states. It thus aims to provide an overall summary measure of quality of life that integrates subjective function states, preferences for these states, morbidity, and mortality.

Cost/Utility Versus Cost/Benefit

The terms *cost/utility, cost/effectiveness,* and *cost/benefit* are used inconsistently in the medical literature (Doubelet, Weinstein, & McNeil, 1986). Some economists have favored the assessment of cost/benefit. These approaches measure both program costs and treatment outcomes in dollar units. For example, treatment outcomes are evaluated in relation to changes in use of medical services, economic productivity, etc. Treatments are cost/beneficial if the economic return exceeds treatment costs. Diabetic patients who are aggressively treated, for example, may need fewer medical services. The savings associated with decreased services might exceed treatment costs. As Kaplan and Davis (1986) argued, there is relatively little strong empirical evidence that patient education or behavioral treatments are actually cost/beneficial. In addition, as suggested by Russell (1986), the requirement that health care treatments reduce costs may be unrealistic. Patients are willing to pay for improvements in health status just as they are willing to pay for other desirable goods and services. We do not treat cancer in order to save money. Instead, treatments are given in order to achieve better health outcomes.

Cost/effectiveness is an alternative approach in which the unit of outcome is a reflection of treatment effect. In recent years, cost/effectiveness has gained considerable attention. Some approaches, such as those advocated by Yates (1978), emphasize simple, treatment-specific outcomes. For example, Yates considers the cost per pound lost as a measure of cost/effectiveness of weight loss programs (e.g., public competitions achieve a lower cost-per-pound loss ratio than do traditional clinical interventions). The major difficulty with cost/effectiveness methodologies is that they do not allow for comparison across very different treatment interventions. For example, health care administrators often need to choose between investments in very different alternatives. They may need to decide between supporting liver transplantation for a few patients versus prenatal counseling for a large number of patients. For the same cost, they may achieve a large effect for a few people or a small effect for a large number of people. The treatment-specific outcomes used in cost/effectiveness studies do not permit these comparisons.

Cost/utility approaches use the expressed preference or utility of a treatment effect as the unit of outcome. As noted in World Health Organization documents (WHO, 1984), the goals of health care are to add years to life and to add life to years. In other words, health care is designed to make people live longer (increase their life expectancy) and to live a higher quality of life in the years prior to death. Cost/utility studies use outcome measures that combine mortality outcomes with quality of life measurements. The utilities are the expressed preferences for observable states of function on a continuum bounded by zero for death to 1.0 for optimum function (Kaplan, 1985a, 1985b; Kaplan & Anderson, 1988a, 1988b; Kaplan & Bush, 1982). In recent years, cost/utility approaches have gained increasing acceptance as methods for comparing many diverse options in health care (Russell, 1986; Weinstein & Stason, 1977; Williams, 1988). The purpose of the General Health Policy Model, to be described in the next section, is to evaluate different health care alternatives using common outcome units.

A General Health Policy Model

Cost studies have gained in popularity because health care costs have grown rapidly in recent years. Not all health care interventions are equally efficient in returning benefit for the expended dollar. Objective cost studies might guide policy makers toward an optimal and equitable distribution of scarce resources. Cost/utility analysis typically quantifies the benefits of a health care intervention in terms of years of life, or *Quality Adjusted Life Years* (QALYs). Cost/utility is a special use of cost/effectiveness that weights observable health states by preferences or utility judgments of quality (Kaplan & Bush, 1982). In cost/utility analysis, the benefits of medical care, behavioral interventions, or preventive programs are expressed in terms of well-years. These outcomes have also been described as QALYs (Weinstein & Stason, 1977), discounted life years (Kaplan, Bush, & Berry, 1976), or health years of life (Russell, 1986). Since the term quality adjusted life years has become most popular, we will use it in this presentation. QALYs integrate mortality and morbidity to express health status in terms of equivalents of well-years of life.

If a man dies of heart disease at age 50 and we would have expected him to live to age 75, it might be concluded that the disease was associated with 25 lost life years. If 100 men died at age 50 (and also had a life expectancy of 75 years) we might conclude that 2,500 (100 men × 25 years) life years had been lost. Yet, death is not the only outcome of concern in heart disease. Many adults suffer myocardial infarctions that leave them somewhat disabled over long periods of time. Although they are still alive, the quality of their lives has diminished. Quality adjusted life years take into consideration the quality of life consequences of these illnesses. For example, a disease that reduces quality of life by one half will take away .5 QALYs over the course of each year. If it affects two people, it will take away 1.0 year (equal 2 × .5) over each year period. A medical treatment that improves quality of life by .2 for each of five individuals will result in the equivalent of one QALY if the benefit is maintained over a one-year period. This system has the advantage of considering both benefits and side-effects of programs in terms of the common QALY units.

The need to integrate mortality and quality of life information is clearly apparent in studies of heart disease. Consider the case of high cholesterol. People with high cholesterol may live shorter lives if they are untreated. Thus, one benefit of treatment is to add years to life. However, for most patients, high cholesterol is not associated with symptoms for many years. Conversely, the treatment for high cholesterol may cause a variety of symptoms. In other words, in the short run, patients taking medication may experience more symptoms than those who avoid it. If a treatment is evaluated only in terms of changes in life expectancy, the benefits of the program will be overestimated because side-effects are not taken into consideration. On the other hand, considering only current quality of life will underestimate the treatment benefits because information on mortality is excluded. In fact, considering only current function might make the treatment look harmful because the side-effects of the treatment might be worse than the symptoms of elevated cholesterol. A comprehensive measurement system may take into consideration side-effects and benefits and provide an overall estimate of the benefit of treatment (Russell, 1986).

Although there are several different approaches for obtaining quality adjusted life years, most of them are similar (Kaplan, 1985b). The approach that our group prefers involves several steps. First, patients are classified according to objective levels of functioning. These levels are represented by scales of mobility, physical activity, and social activity. The dimensions and steps for these levels of functioning are shown in Table 1. Note that these steps are not actually the scale, only listings of labels representing the scale steps. Standardized questionnaires have been developed to classify individuals into one of each of these scale steps (Anderson, Bush, & Berry, 1986). In addition to classification into these observable levels of function, individuals are also classified by the one symptom or problem that bothered them most (see Table 2). About half of the population reports at least one symptom on any day. Symptoms may be severe, such as serious chest pain, or minor, such as the inconvenience of taking medication or a prescribed diet for health reasons. The functional classification (Table 1) and the accompanying list of symptoms or problems (Table 2) were created after extensive reviews of the medical and public health literature (Kaplan, Bush, & Berry, 1976). Over the last decade, the function classification system and symptom list were repeatedly shortened until we arrived at the current versions. With structured questionnaires, an interviewer can obtain classifications on these dimensions in 11 to 16 minutes.

Once observable behavioral levels of functioning have been classified, a second step is required to place each individual on the 0 to 1.0 scale of well-

TABLE 1 Quality of well-being general health policy model and sample calculation

Step no.	Step definition	Weight
Mobility scale (MOB)		
5	No limitations for health reasons	−0.000
4	Did not drive a car, health related: did not ride in a car as usual for age (15 yr) (health related), *and/or* did not use public transportation (health related), *or* had or would have used more help than usual for age to use public transportation (health related)	−0.062
2	In hospital, health related	−0.090
Physical activity scale (PAC)		
4	No limitations for health reasons	−0.000
3	In wheelchair, moved or controlled movement of wheelchair without help from someone else, *or* had trouble or did not try to lift, stoop, bend over, or use stairs or inclines (health related) *and/or* limped, used a cane, crutches, or walker (health related), *and/or* had any other physical limitation in walking, or did not try to walk as far or as fast as others the same age are able (health related)	−0.060
1	In wheelchair, did not move or control the movement of wheelchair without help from someone else, *or* in bed, chair, or couch for most or all of the day (health related)	−0.077
Social activity scale (SAC)		
5	No limitations for health reasons	−0.000
4	Limited in other (e.g., recreational) role activity (health related)	−0.061
3	Limited in major (primary) role activity (health related)	−0.061
2	Performed no major role activity (health related) but did perform self-care activities	−0.061
1	Performed no major role (health related) *and* did not perform or had more trouble than usual in performance of one or more self-care activities (health related)	−0.106

Calculating formulas

Formula 1: Point-in-time well-being score for an individual (W):

$$W = 1 + (CPXwt + MOBwt) + PACwt + SAC\ wt$$

where wt is the preference-weighted measure for each factor and CPX is the symptom/problem complex. For example, the W score for a person with the following description profile may be calculated for one day as follows:

TABLE 1 Quality of well-being general health policy model and sample calculation (*Continued*)

Quality of well-being element	Step definition	Weight
CPX-11	Cough, wheezing, or shortness of breath, with or without fever, chills, or aching all over	−0.257
MOB-5	No limitations	−0.000
PAC-1	In bed, chair, or couch for most or all of day (health related)	−0.077
SAC-2	Performed no major role activity (health related) but did perform self-care	−0.061

$$W = 1 + -0.257 + -0.000 + -0.007 + -0.061 = 0.605$$

Formula 2: Well years (WY) as an output measure:

$$WY = [\text{No. of persons} \times (\text{CPXwt} + \text{MOBwt} + \text{PACwt} + \text{SACwt})] \times \text{time}$$

Note. From Kaplan, R. M., and Anderson, J. P. (1988b). Reprinted by permission.

ness. To accomplish this, the observable health states are weighted by "quality" ratings for the desirability of these conditions. Human value studies have been conducted to place the observable states onto a preference continuum, with an anchor of 0 for death and 1.0 for completely well. In several studies, random samples of citizens from a metropolitan community evaluated the desirability of over 400 case descriptions. Using these ratings, a preference structure that assigns weights to each combination of an observable state and a symptom/problem has been developed (Kaplan et al., 1976). Cross validation studies have shown that the model can be used to assign weights to other states of functioning with a high degree of accuracy ($R^2 = .96$). The regression weights obtained in these studies are given in Tables 1 and 2. Studies have shown that the weights are highly stable over a 1-year period and that they are consistent across diverse groups of raters (Kaplan, Bush, & Berry, 1978). Finally, it is necessary to consider the duration of stay in various health states. For example, one year in a state that has been assigned the weight of .5 is equivalent to .5 of a QALY. Table 1 provides an illustrative example of calculation.

The well life expectancy is the current life expectancy adjusted for diminished quality of life associated with dysfunctional states and duration of stay in each state. Using the system, it is possible to simultaneously consider mortality, morbidity, and the preference weights for these observable behavioral states of function. When the proper steps have been followed, the model quantifies the health activity or treatment program in terms of the QALYs that it produces or saves. A QALY is defined conceptually as the equivalent of a completely well year of life, or a year of life free of any symptoms, problems, or health-related disabilities.

More detailed descriptions of this system are available in other publications

TABLE 2 List of quality of well-being general health policy model symptom/problem complexes (CPX) with calculating weights

CPX no.	CPX description	Weights
1	Death (not on respondent's card)	−0.727
2	Loss of consciousness such as seizure (fits), fainting, or coma ("out cold" or "knocked out")	−0.407
3	Burn over large areas of face, body, arms or legs	−0.387
4	Pain, bleeding, itching, or discharge (drainage) from sexual organs—does not include normal menstrual bleeding	−0.349
5	Trouble learning, remembering, or thinking clearly	−0.340
6	Any combination of one or more hands, feet, arms, or legs either missing, deformed (crooked), paralyzed (unable to move), or broken—includes wearing artificial limbs or braces	−0.333
7	Pain, stiffness, weakness, numbness, or other discomfort in chest, stomach (including hernia or rupture), side, neck, back, hips, or any joints or hands, feet, arms, or legs	−0.299
8	Pain, burning, bleeding, itching, or other difficulty with rectum, bowel movements, or urination (passing water)	−0.292
9	Sick or upset stomach, vomiting, or loose bowel movement, with or without fever, chills, or aching all over	−0.290
10	General tiredness, weakness, or weight loss	−0.259
11	Cough, wheezing, or shortness of breath with or without fever, chills, or aching all over	−0.257
12	Spells of feeling upset, being depressed, or crying	−0.257
13	Headache, dizziness, ringing in ears, or spells of feeling hot, nervous, or shaky	−0.244
14	Burning or itching rash on large areas of face, body, arms, or legs	−0.240
15	Trouble talking such as lisp, stuttering, hoarseness, or being unable to speak	−0.227
16	Pain or discomfort in one or both eyes (such as burning or itching) or any trouble seeing after correction	−0.230
17	Overweight for age and height or skin defect of face, body, arms, or legs such as scars, pimples, warts, bruises, or changes in color	−0.188
18	Pain in ear, tooth, jaw, throat, lips, tongue: several missing or crooked permanent teeth—includes wearing bridges or false teeth; stuffy, runny nose; or any trouble hearing—includes wearing a hearing aid	−0.170
19	Taking medication or staying on a prescribed diet for health reasons	−0.144
20	Wore eyeglasses or contact lenses	−0.101
21	Breathing smog or unpleasant air	−0.101
22	No symptoms or problem (not on respondent's card)	−0.000
23	Standard symptom/problem	−0.257

Note. From Kaplan, R. M., and Anderson, J. P. (1988b). Reprinted by permission.

(Kaplan, 1985a, 1985b; Kaplan & Bush, 1982). In the following sections, we will illustrate applications of the QALY concept.

Health Promotion

Health promotion is the effort to ensure a healthy population through disease prevention and the promotion of health lifestyles. Health promotion has now become a major growth industry. Weight control alone may be a billion dollar industry. Health promotion involves not only the use of behavioral interventions, but also the use of food and drug interventions. In 1986, three of the ten most widely used drugs in the world (Tenormin, Inderal, and Aldomet) were products to lower blood pressure (Rukeyser & Cooney, 1988). One of the most important justifications for health promotion programs is that they reduce health care costs. Yet several authors have begun to challenge the cost/effectiveness of prevention or health promotion programs. In an intriguing book, Russell (1986) posed the challenging question, *Is Prevention Better Than Cure?* Weinstein (1986) suggested that the belief in health promotion as a money saving venture was "naive assumption number one." More recently Warner, Wickizer, Wolfe, Schildroth, and Samuelson (1988) examined the conventional wisdom that work place health promotion programs yield financial dividends for companies. After reviewing the literature, they concluded that most studies published prior to 1986 did conclude that health promotion programs increased profitability. However, these studies tended to use anecdotal evidence for analyses that were seriously flawed in terms of their assumptions or methodology. In fact, they found very little evidence that health promotion programs save money for companies. However, they also found little evidence against this assertion. The difficulty was that few studies had systematically examined the issue. Thus, they recommended healthy skepticism for readers of the literature. In the next sections we will review the evidence for the cost/effectiveness of interventions to lower cholesterol and to reduce cigarette smoking. The economic incentives for achieving these changes varies. In each case, the outcomes will be conceptualized in terms of years of life or well-years gained.

Industry and Health Outcomes

There is considerable commercial interest in promoting health. Indeed, many products and services are offered because they can enhance health status. Food is one of the most interesting of these commercial interests. Each year, Americans spend about $513 billion on food and beverages (about the same as they spend on health care). About $10 billion is spent on health enhancing activities, such as diet food, health clubs, diet drugs, and weight reduction programs. We spend about $800 million on frozen dinners that may not be nutritious and then devote about $350 million to diet pills and diet powders. Weight Watchers

International, one of many weight reduction programs, has had 25 million participants with 700,000 currently enrolled. The value of the company is estimated to be about $400 million in gross receipts (Rukeyser & Cooney, 1988).

An example of the commercialization of health promotion is provided by the February 13, 1989 issue of *Newsweek.* Each year, *Newsweek* magazine provides a supplement, typically written by physicians, on health promotion. This particular supplement focused on heart health. The supplement included five articles. Adjacent to each page of the supplement was a full-page ad for a commercial product. The table of contents faced an ad for Bayer aspirin. Recent evidence has suggested that regular use of aspirin may reduce the probability of a fatal myocardial infarction. However, these same studies show no advantage of aspirin for increasing survival because reductions in heart attacks are associated with increases in other types of cardiovascular death (Kaplan, 1989). The first article on heart attack prevention was followed by a two-page advertisement for Kellogg's Oat Bran. The two-page article on exercise included two one-page advertisements, one for Schwinn Fitness Machines (stationary bicycles) and another for Nordic track stationary cross-country machines. The third article was on healthy eating. It was two pages long and was accompanied by two full-page advertisements, one for Metamucil, a bulk laxative that was promoted as a good source of wheat and oat bran, and an advertisement for Miracle Whip, which was promoted as a healthier product than mayonnaise. There was then an article on exercise, followed by another full page ad for Kellogg's Oat Bran. Then, there was an article on what to do about a heart attack accompanied by a full page ad for Tylenol. The Tylenol ad acknowledged that many people are now taking aspirin to prevent a heart attack. The ad read, "If you are taking aspirin for your heart, you probably shouldn't take aspirin for your headache." The section ended with a full-page advertisement for Searle Pharmaceuticals. In total, the 20-page supplement included 10 full pages of advertising. Remarkably, the 20-page supplement on prevention of heart attacks devotes only two paragraphs to cigarette smoking, even though cigarette smoking is clearly the most important modifiable risk factor for coronary heart disease. On the back cover of that particular issue of *Newsweek*, somewhat far away from the healthy heart supplement, was a full-page, full-color advertisement for Marlboro cigarettes.

In the next sections, we will review the rationale for two different approaches to health promotion. One approach involves lowering cholesterol and the other requires reducing the use of cigarettes. The two approaches will be compared using concepts relevant to cost/utility analysis.

Cholesterol

Coronary heart disease remains the major cause of death in the United States. In fact, heart disease still accounts for nearly half of fatalities. Upon review of the evidence, a National Institutes of Health (1985) Consensus Conference concluded that lowering cholesterol levels will significantly reduce deaths from cardiovascular diseases. Thus, major efforts toward cholesterol reduction have been stimulated. In previous papers, I have challenged the notion that reductions in mortality can be easily achieved through health promotion programs designed to reduce dietary cholesterol (Kaplan, 1984, 1985a).

Evidence that serum cholesterol is related to mortality has been provided in several studies. For example, Stamler, Wentworth, and Neaton (1986) presented mortality data from over 350,000 men whose cholesterol had been measured as part of the Multiple Risk Factors Intervention Trial (MRFIT). When these men were followed prospectively, there was a systematic relationship between level of elevation and blood cholesterol and likelihood of dying from heart disease.

Many health promotion programs emphasize change in dietary habits. Since cholesterol builds up in the arteries, many people assume that avoiding foods with cholesterol will reduce the chances of developing heart problems. Thus, many advertisements emphasize that particular foods have no cholesterol. However, the direct relationship between serum cholesterol and dietary cholesterol has been difficult to demonstrate. Some studies have shown that the *mean* serum cholesterol level is higher in countries where, on the average, high levels of fat are consumed, and the *mean* level of cholesterol is lower in countries where lower levels of cholesterol are consumed. Yet, correlational studies within each of these cultures often fail to show significant associations between cholesterol consumption and serum cholesterol. There are many different explanations for this failure to find an association between dietary cholesterol and serum cholesterol. For example, some authors have suggested that serum cholesterol is primarily influenced by genetic factors (Steinberg, 1979). Others suggest that a significant true correlation may be disguised because of measurement error in the assessment of dietary habits (Jacobs, Anderson, & Blackburn, 1979). Attenuation caused by this measurement error obscures potential true correlation. However, this possible explanation for a nonsignificant correlation does not mean that the significant correlation exists.

Perhaps the most pessimistic view of the cholesterol evidence has been presented by Stallones (1983). Using data from six prospective American epidemiologic studies and one British study, Stallones reported that those who die of heart disease do not consume more calories, more fat, or more cholesterol than those who remain well. Indeed, the evidence on dietary cholesterol is difficult to interpret. Studies conducted in metabolic wards clearly do demonstrate that reductions in the consumption of dietary cholesterol and dietary saturated fat result in reductions in serum cholesterol. In addition, animal studies also demonstrate the cholesterol-lowering benefits of dietary manipulation. Yet, there is very little evidence showing the long-term benefits of dietary manipulation in humans.

In previous papers, we have reviewed the experimental trials on cholesterol reduction. This is a complex literature and one that is difficult to interpret. Recently, for example, six cholesterol-lowering studies were critically evaluated (Kaplan, 1988). Several of these studies have demonstrated that lowering blood cholesterol results in reductions in coronary heart disease deaths. However, in each of these studies there is an unexpected finding for total deaths. Mortality averaged over all causes of death is typically not affected by the dietary interventions. Reductions in deaths from heart disease are usually associated with increases in deaths from other causes.

Perhaps the most influential study on cholesterol lowering was the National Heart, Lung, and Blood Institute Coronary Primary Prevention Trial (Lipid Research Clinics Program, 1984). This randomized experimental trial assigned high-risk men to either a placebo or cholestyramine, a drug that is known to reduce serum cholesterol levels significantly. Long-term follow-up was conducted over 10-year period to determine differential mortalities from heart disease in the two groups. Cholestyramine was successful in lowering cholesterol by an average of 8.5% in the treatment group. Those in the treatment group experienced 24% fewer heart disease deaths and 19% fewer heart attacks than the placebo group. As in other studies, differences between the groups for total mortality were not statistically significant.

Although the results of the coronary primary prevention trial are very important, it is not clear that they are directly relevant to most health promotion efforts. Many authors assume that the results apply directly to diet. In fact, the subjects in the experimental all have failed to respond to dietary intervention prior to assignment into cholestyramine or placebo groups. Preliminary analysis in the CPPT trial failed to reveal any significant benefits of dietary intervention. Another feature of the CPPT trial was that it was directed to those at the extreme of the cholesterol distribution. In order to be included as a subject, a male participant had to be above the 95th percentile in serum cholesterol. The results tell us very little about diet or cholestyramine for those who did not have significantly elevated cholesterol. Even for those at high risk, the results may be difficult to understand. Although there was a 24% reduction in mortality in the treated group, the actual percentage of patients who died was similar in the two groups. In the placebo group, there were 38 deaths among 1,900 participants (2%). In the cholestyramine group, there were 30 deaths among 1,906 participants (1.6%). Thus, over a 7- to 10-year period, the medication reduced the chances of dying from 2% to 1.6%. Again, it is important to emphasize that this difference (.4%) refers to the chances of dying from heart disease. The cholestyramine group actually had higher chances of dying from other diseases. Thus, there was no difference whatsoever in total deaths. At the end of the study, 3.7% of those in the placebo group had died, while 3.6% of those in the cholestyramine group had died. The successful intervention changed the cause of death but not the total number of people who died or survived.

Despite some of the confusion about cholesterol reduction, it has become apparent that cholesterol management is a national objective. This has been recommended by the National Institutes of Health (1985) Consensus Panel and has stimulated a growth industry of cholesterol lowering products.

One of the issues in the attempt to find methods to lower cholesterol has been the cost to achieve significant changes in health outcome. Several policy analyses have warned that cholesterol reduction will be a valuable but expensive way to promote health outcomes (Oster & Epstein, 1987; Weinstein & Stason, 1985; Himmelstein & Woolhandler, 1984). However, the high cost estimates may have resulted because the method for lowering cholesterol was an expensive cholesterol lowering drug such as cholestyramine resin. There are several alternative treatments for high cholesterol that might produce effective cholesterol lowering at a fraction of the cost. These methods have recently been compared by Kinosian and Eisenberg (1988).

In the Kinosian and Eisenberg simulation, three different approaches to cholesterol lowering were considered. The first approach involved the use of cholestyramine resin. Cholestyramine binds bile acids and blocks the endogenous production of cholesterol. A similar product, cholestopol, has equivalent effects but is offered at a lower cost. These two products were used in the analysis and were considered in two different ways. Since the products are often offered by prescription only, there is a considerable difference between retail price and bulk price. Both of these are considered in the analysis. For comparison, oat bran was also considered. There is growing evidence that oat bran, taken in substantial doses (60 to 90 g/day, or the equivalent 1 to 1.5 cups/day) can reduce serum cholesterol by 13% to 19% (Anderson, Story, Sieling, et al., 1984).

The results of the Kinosian and Eisenberg analyses are summarized in Figure 1. As the figure suggests, there are savings in cost/year of life saved for buying either cholestyramine or cholestopol in bulk. However, the most striking aspect of the figure is that oat bran produces years of life saved at a cost much less than either of the prescription medications. On a population basis, nonprescription oat bran may be the most cost-effective alternative.

We must now tackle the difficult question of whether or not investing in cholesterol lowering has advantages relative to other investments in prevention. Investments in programs to reduce cigarette smoking or to prevent cigarette smoking will be considered to illustrate this point.

Cigarette Smoking

It has now been one quarter of a century since the publication of the surgeon general's first report, *Smoking and health: Report of the advisory committee to the surgeon general of the United States* (U.S. Public Health Service, 1964). Twenty-five years ago there was strong evidence for the detrimental effects of

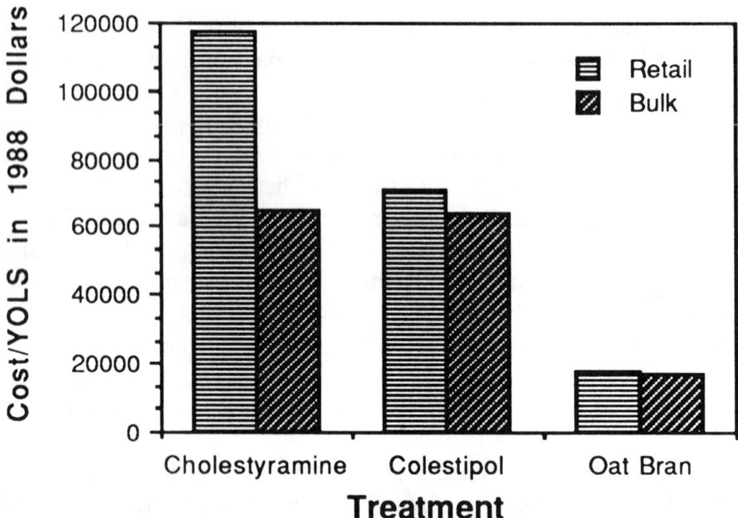

FIGURE 1 Comparison of three approaches to cholesterol lowering in terms of cost per year of life saved (YOLS). Data from Kinosian and Eisenberg (1988).

cigarette smoking. Current evidence on the health consequences of cigarette smoking leaves no doubt that cigarettes cause premature deaths. According to the American Cancer Society, 390,000 people in the United States died of cigarette smoking in 1985. That is one fifth of all deaths in the United States! (American Cancer Society, 1988). Many of our public health programs are directed toward preventing the most feared types of death. Enormous amounts of public attention are devoted to AIDS, cocaine, heroin, homicide, and suicide. However, it is important to emphasize that the impact of cigarette smoking far exceeds that for any of these other causes of death. In fact, cigarette smoking causes more premature deaths than the combination of AIDS, cocaine, heroin, alcohol, fire, automobile accidents, homicide, and suicide (Warner, 1987). Thirty percent of all cancer deaths are caused by cigarette smoking, as are 21% of all cases of coronary heart disease death. Stroke, a disabling disease, is also closely linked to the use of cigarettes. An overwhelming 82% of deaths from chronic obstructive pulmonary disease (chronic bronchitis and emphysema) are attributable to cigarette smoking (American Cancer Society, 1988).

The epidemic of deaths associated with cigarette use is directly traceable to investments by tobacco companies in advertising. Groups are targeted and advertising material is directed toward them. There is substantial evidence that cigarette smoking rates increase in these targeted groups. Women, for example, are a major new target of cigarette advertising and lung cancer is now a major cause of death for women. Twenty-five years ago, lung cancer was a relatively uncommon disease in women. Over the last twenty-five years, lung cancer rates for nonsmoking women have remained constant at about 12/100,000 women. For smoking women, lung cancer death rates rose from 23.9/100,000 to 130.4/100,000 (USDHHS, 1989). Lung cancer alone is the major factor affecting the increasing rate of deaths from cancer. In fact, age-adjusted non-lung cancer death rates have actually been falling, and we would have a declining rate of cancer death if it were not for cigarette smoking.

In addition to targeting women, the tobacco industry is also focusing on young children, minorities, and third world countries. As Warner argued in a recent editorial (Warner, 1989) we are rapidly exporting our epidemic to third world countries. It is ironic that the U.S. government is outraged that some countries have been involved in the export of cocaine to the United States. Yet at the same time, federal policies actually encourage American companies to export deadly tobacco products. Indeed, the toll in death and suffering from tobacco availability exceed that for the availability of cocaine.

Although the tobacco industry argues that they do not market cigarettes to children and adolescents, substantial evidence demonstrates the opposite. Ads for tobacco products are consistently placed in publications that are distributed primarily to the young. Indeed, the tobacco habit typically starts in youth. Ninety percent of all cigarette smokers began before the age of 19 years and 60% started by the age of 14 years. Tobacco is highly addictive, and once "hooked," cigarette smokers have great difficulty breaking the habit (USDHHS, 1989).

Several investigators have attempted to simulate the impact of smoking cessation and smoking prevention. In one analysis, Oster, Huse, Delea, and Colditz (1986) examined the cost-effectiveness of using Nicotine gum in addition to a physician's advice against cigarette smoking. They estimated that the cost to save a year of life with smoking cessation was about $4,000 dollars. This was considerably below a wide variety of other popular prevention efforts. In another analysis, Taylor, Pass, Shepard, and Komaroff (1987) compared three different approaches to prevention. Cholesterol reduction, blood pressure reduction, and smoking prevention. They assumed that cholesterol could be lowered 6.7% with a dietary intervention because that was what was achieved in the Multiple Risk Factors Intervention Trial (MRFIT, 1982). They also assumed that blood pressure could be reduced 15%, because that was the level achieved in the Hypertension and Detection Follow-up Program (HDFP, 1979). Then, they estimated the years of life added by smoking cessation for smokers or total prevention of cigarette use. The analysis was done separately for men and women, assuming that the treatment began at age 20, 40, or 60. Figure 2 summarizes the Taylor analysis. As the figure suggests, cholesterol reduction has very little impact on life expectancy, particularly if it begins at age 60. In fact, cholesterol reduction programs may add only about 2 months of life for 60-year-old men. The benefits of blood pressure reduction are intermediate and have the most dramatic effects if the program for men begins early in life. Most striking is the impact of programs for cigarette smoking. As the figure demonstrates, prevention of cigarette use adds a full five years of life if smoking is prevented before age 20. Clearly, not all health promotion programs yield the same benefits.

Figure 3 is adapted from the Kinosian and Eisenberg (1988) analysis. The figure compares the cost per year of life gained for a variety of treatments and preventive efforts relevant to coronary heart disease. As the figure demonstrates, the cost per year of life saved with cigarette smoking is much less than it is for cholesterol lowering or for surgery. For the cholesterol lowering options, the nontraditional, nondiagnosis related approach using oat bran is more cost-effective than the other alternatives.

CONCLUSION

In this chapter, we have considered several different approaches to prevention. Preventing heart attack deaths through cholesterol lowering is an important

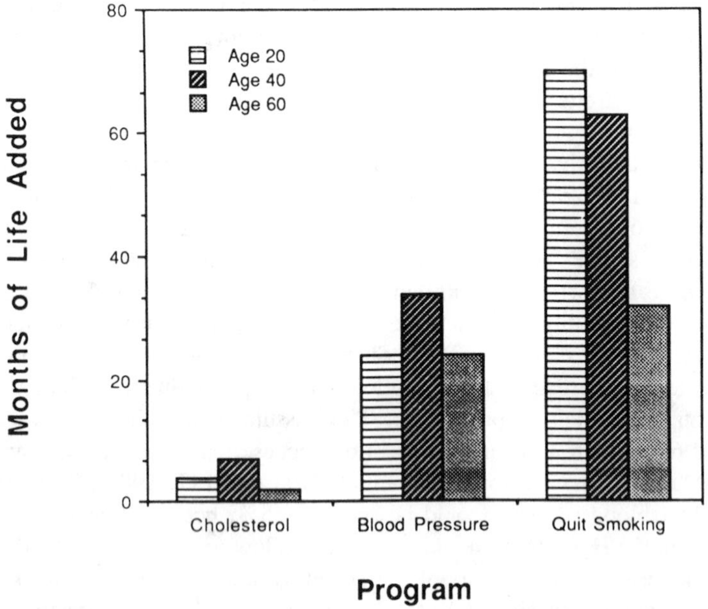

FIGURE 2 Months of life added by three different health promotion efforts, for men beginning programs at age 20, 40, or 60 years. Data from Taylor et al. (1987).

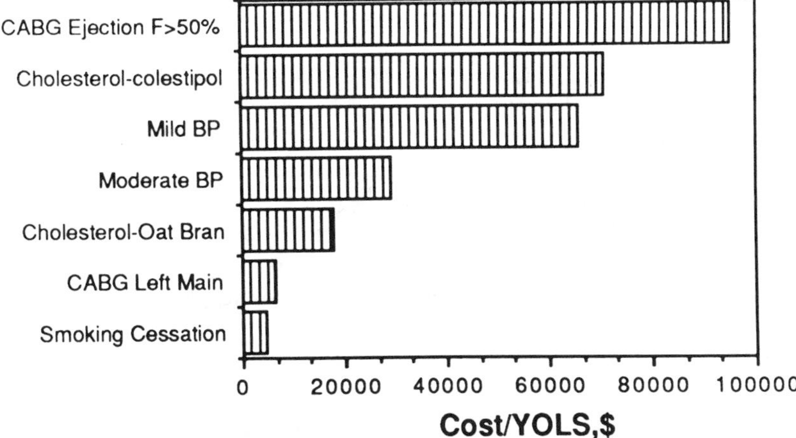

FIGURE 3 Comparison of options to treat coronary heart disease in terms of cost per year of life saved (YOLS). Data from Kinosian and Eisenberg (1988). Adapted by permission. CABG, coronary artery bypass graft surgery; Ejection F, heart ejection fraction; Mild BP, screening for and treatment of mild high blood pressure, defined as diastolic > 95 mm Hg < 104 mm Hg; Moderate BP, screening and treatment of moderate high blood pressure, defined as diastolic pressure > 105 mm Hg; CABG left main, coronary artery bypass surgery for patients with occlusion of the left main artery.

approach, and one that has traditional economic advocates. There are strong financial incentives to use the traditional health care system to diagnose problems and to treat those problems using medications. Using a general health policy model, it is suggested that nontraditional approaches in which all citizens make dietary changes may be a more cost-effective approach to this problem. The most expensive approach may not necessarily be the most effective approach and is usually not the most cost-effective approach.

Not all approaches to prevention are equally useful. As this analysis has shown, investing in smoking cessation and smoking prevention yields many more benefits than do interventions to change cholesterol. Yet it is more difficult to make money preventing smoking or changing smoking habits than it is to diagnose diseases and treat them using medications. Thus, smoking cessation has fewer economic advocates than does treatment of blood pressure or cholesterol. Further, there is a strong lobby actively promoting the use of cigarettes and other tobacco products.

A general health policy model may contribute to the assessment of these policy problems. The development of the model is in a relatively early stage, and many measurement issues still need to be resolved. Nevertheless, I believe that this approach has promise for clarifying policy alternatives.

REFERENCES

American Cancer Society. (1988). *Cancer: Facts and figures, 1988.* New York: American Cancer Society.

Anderson, J. P., Bush, J. W., & Berry, C. C. (1986). Classifying function for health outcome and quality of life evaluation. Self-versus-interviewer modes. *Medical Care, 24,* 454–469.

Anderson, J. W., Story, L., Sieling, B., Chen, W. J., Petro, M. S. Story, J. (1984). Hypocholesterolemic effects of oat-bran or bean intake for hypercholesterolemic men. *American Journal of Clinical Nutrition,* 40, 1146–1155.

Bergner, M. (1985). Measurement of health status. *Medical Care, 23,* 696–704.

Bergner, M., Bobbitt, R. A., Carter, W. B., & Gilson, B. S. (1981). The sickness impact profile: Development and final revision of a health status measure. *Medical Care, 19,* 787–805.

Bush, J. W. (1984). Relative preferences versus relative frequencies in health-related quality of life evaluations. In N. K. Wenger, M. E. Mattson, C. D. Furberg, & J. Elinson (Eds.), *Assessment of quality of life in clinical trails of cardiovascular therapies* (pp. 118–139). New York: LaJacq Publishing Company.

Croog, S. H., Levine, S., Testa, M. A., Brown, D., Bulpitt, C. J., Jenkins, C. D., Klerman, G. L., & Williams, G. H. (1986). The effects of anti-hypertensive therapy on quality of life. *New England Journal of Medicine, 314,* 1657–1664.

Doubelet, P., Weinstein, M. C., & McNeil, B. J. (1986). Use and misuse of the term "cost/effectiveness" in medicine. *New England Journal of Medicine, 314,* 253–256.

Follick, M. J., Gorkin, L., Smith, T., Capone, R. J., & Stabein, D. (1988). Quality of life post-myocardial infarction: Effects of a transtelephonic coronary intervention system. *Health Psychology, 7,* 169–182.

Galbraith, J. K. (1958). *The affluent society.* Boston: Houghton Mifflin.

Himmelstein, D., & Woolhandler, S. (1984). Free care, cholestyramine, and health policy. *New England Journal of Medicine, 311,* 1511–1514.

Hunt, S. M., & McEwen, J. (1983). The development of a subjective health indicator. *Sociology of Health and Illness, 2,* 231–245.

Hypertension Detection and Follow-up Program Cooperative Group. (1979). Five-year findings of hypertension detection and follow-up programs: Reduction in mortality of persons with high blood pressure, including mild hypertension. *Journal of the American Medical Association, 242,* 2562–2571.

Jacobs, D. R., Anderson, J. T., & Blackburn, H. (1979). Diet and serum cholesterol: Do zero correlations negate the relationship? *American Journal of Epidemiology, 110,* 77–87.

Kaplan, R. M. (1984). The connection between clinical health promotion and health status: A critical review. *American Psychologist, 39,* 755–765.

Kaplan, R. M. (1985a). Behavioral epidemiology, health promotion, and health services. *Medical Care, 23,* 564–583.

Kaplan, R. M. (1985b). Quantification of health outcomes for policy studies in behavioral epidemiology. In R. M. Kaplan & M. H. Criqui (Eds.), *Behavioral epidemiology and disease prevention* (pp. 31–54). New York: Plenum.

Kaplan, R. M. (1988). The value dimension in studies of health promotion. In S. Spacapan & S. Oskamp (Eds.), *The social psychology of health* (pp. 207–236). Beverly Hills: Sage Publications.

Kaplan, R. M. (1989). Models of health outcome for policy analysis. *Health Psychology,* 8, 723–735.

Kaplan, R. M., & Anderson, J. P. (1988a). A general health policy model: Update and applications. *Health Services Research, 23,* 203–235.

Kaplan, R. M., & Anderson, J. P. (1988b). The quality of well-being scale: Rationale for a single quality of life index. In S. R. Walker & R. Rosser (Eds.), *Quality of life: Assessment and applications* (pp. 51–77). London: MTP Press.

Kaplan, R. M., & Bush, J. W. (1982). Health-related quality of life measurement for evaluation research and policy analysis. *Health Psychology, 1,* 61–80.

Kaplan, R. M., Bush, J. W., & Berry, C. C. (1976). Health status: Types of validity for an index of well-being. *Health Services Research, 11,* 478–507.

Kaplan, R. M., Bush, J. W., & Berry, C. C. (1978). The reliability, stability, and generalizability of a health index. *American Statistical Association, Proceedings of the Social Statistics Section,* 704–708.

Kaplan, R. M., & Davis, W. K. (1986). Evaluating the costs and benefits of outpatient diabetes education and nutritional counseling. *Diabetes Care, 9,* 81–86.

Kinosian, B. P., & Eisenberg, J. M. (1988). Cutting into cholesterol: Cost/effectiveness alternatives for treating hypercholesterolemia. *Journal of the American Medical Association, 259,* 2249–2254.

Lipid Research Clinics Program. (1984). The Lipid Research Clinics primary coronary prevention trial results: I. Reduction in the incidence of coronary heart disease. *Journal of the American Medical Association, 253,* 351–364.

National Center for Health Statistics. (1986). *Current estimates from the National Health Interview Survey.* Washington, DC: U.S. Department of Health and Human Services.

National Institutes of Health. (1979). *Epidemiology of Respiratory Diseases*

Task Force (NIH Publication No. 81:2019). Washington, DC: U.S. Government Printing Office.

National Institutes of Health. (1985). Lowering Blood Cholesterol to Prevent Heart Disease, Consensus Conference. *Journal of the American Medical Association, 253,* 2080–2086.

Oster, G., & Epstein, A. (1987). The cost/effectiveness of antihyperlipidemic therapy in the prevention of coronary heart disease: The case of cholestyramine. *Journal of the American Medical Association, 258,* 2381–2387.

Oster, G., Huse, D. M., Delea, T. E., and Colditz, G. A. (1986). Cost/effectiveness of nicotine gum as an adjunct to physician's advice against cigarette smoking. *Journal of the American Medical Association, 256,* 1315–1318.

Rice, R. M. (1984). Organizational work and the overall quality of life. In S. Oskamp (Ed.), *Applied Social Psychology Annual: Applications in Organizational Settings* (Vol. 5, pp. 155–178). Beverly Hills, CA: Sage.

Rimm, A. A. (1985). Trends in cardiac surgery in the United States. *New England Journal of Medicine, 312,* 119–120.

Rokeach, M. (1973). *The nature of human values.* New York: The Free Press.

Roos, N. P. (1984). Hysterectomy: Variations in rates across small areas and across physicians' practices. *American Journal of Public Health, 74,* 327–355.

Rukeyser, L., & Cooney, J. (1988). *Louis Rukeyser's business almanac.* New York: Simon & Schuster.

Russell, L. (1986). *Is prevention better than cure?* Washington, DC: The Brookings Institution.

Schroeder, S. A. (1987). Strategies for reducing medical costs by changing physicians' behavior. *International Journal of Technology in Health Care, 3,* 39–50.

Sick health services (1988, July 16). *The Economist,* pp. 19–22.

Stallones, R. A. (1983). Ischemic heart disease and lipids in blood and diet. *Annual Review of Nutrition, 3,* 155–185.

Stamler, J., Wentworth, D., & Neaton, J. D. (1986). Is the relationship between serum cholesterol and risk of premature death from coronary heart disease continuous and graded? *Journal of the American Medical Association, 256,* 2823–2828.

Steinberg, D. (1981). Metabolism of lipoproteins at the cellular level in relation to atherogenesis. In N. E. Miller & B. Lewis (Eds.), *Lipoproteins, arthrosclerosis, and coronary heart disease* (pp. 31–48). Amsterdam: Elsevier.

Stewart, A. L., Ware, J. E., Brook, R. H., & Davies-Avery, A. (1978). *Conceptualization and measurement of health for adults: Volume II. Physical health in terms of functioning.* Santa Monica, CA: RAND Corporation.

Taylor, W. C., Pass, T. M., Shepard, D. S., Komaroff, A. L. (1987). Cholesterol reduction and life expectancy: A model incorporating multiple risk factors. *Annals of Internal Medicine, 106,* 605–614.

U.S. Department of Health and Human Services, CDC Office of Smoking and Health. (1989). *Reducing the consequences of smoking: Twenty-five years of progress.* Washington, DC: U.S. Government Printing Office.

U.S. Public Health Service. (1964). *Smoking and health. Report of the Advisory Committee to the Surgeon General of the Public Health Service* (PHS Publication No. 1103). Washington, DC: U.S. Government Printing Office.

Voulgaropolous, D., Schneiderman, L. J., & Kaplan, R. M. (1989). *Recommendations against the use of medical procedures: Evidence, judgment and ethical implications.* Manuscript submitted for publication.

Walker, S., & Rosser, R. (Eds.). (1988). *Quality of life: Assessment and applications.* London: WTP Press.

Warner, K. E. (1987). Health and economic implications of a tobacco-free society. *Journal of the American Medical Association, 258,* 2080–2086.

Warner, K. E. (1989). Smoking and health: A twenty-five year perspective. *American Journal of Public Health, 79,* 141–143.

Warner, K. E., Wickizer, T. M., Wolfe, R. A., Schildroth, J. E., & Samuelson, M. H. (1988). Economic implications of workplace health promotion programs: Review of the literature. *Journal of Occupational Medicine, 30,* 102–112.

Weinstein, M. C. (1986). *How to model health effects: The case of hypertension.* Paper presented at the Workshop on Evaluating Preventive Care, Washington, DC: The Brooks Institute.

Weinstein, M. C., & Stason, W. B. (1977). Foundations of cost/effectiveness analysis for health and medical practice. *New England Journal of Medicine, 296,* 716–721.

Weinstein, M. C., & Stason, W. B. (1985). Cost/effectiveness of interventions to prevent or treat coronary heart disease. *Annual Review of Public Health, 6,* 41–43.

Wenger, N. K., Mattson, M. E., Furberg, C. D., & Elinson, J. (1984). *Assessment of quality of life in clinical trials of cardiovascular therapies.* New York: LaJacq.

Wennberg, J. E. (1990). Small area analysis in the medical care outcome problem. In L. Sechrest, E. Perrin, & J. Bunker (Eds.), *Strengthening causal interpretations of nonexperimental data.* Beverly Hills: Sage.

Wennberg, J. E., Freeman, J. L., & Culp, W. S. (1987). Are health services rationed in New Haven or over utilized in Boston? *Lancet, 23,* 1185–1189.

Williams, A. (1988). The importance of quality of life in policy decisions. In S. Walker & R. Rosser (Eds.), *Quality of life: Assessment and application* (pp. 279–290). London: MTP Press.

World Health Organization. (1948). *Constitution of the World Health Organization.* Geneva: WHO Basic Documents.

World Health Organization. (1984). *Health promotion. A discussion document on the concepts and principles* (unpublished document ICP/HRS 602 (m01). Copenhagen: WHO Regional Office for Europe.

Yates, B. T. (1978). Improving the cost/effectiveness of obesity programs: Three basic strategies for reducing the cost per pound. *International Journal of Obesity, 2*, 249–266.

2

FAMILY SYSTEMS AND HEALTH BEHAVIORS

David H. Olson

University of Minnesota

Kenneth L. Stewart

North Dakota State University

OVERVIEW OF THE FAMILY AND HEALTH BEHAVIORS

This chapter provides an overview of family systems, family assessment, and the impact of the family on health. It reviews family theorists' attempts to collapse the multitude of family system variables into fewer, more integrative system dimensions. These dimensions are then used theoretically to create valid and reliable family assessment instruments.

The family systems paradigm and family assessment have increasingly been used to study the family's impact on physical and mental health, prevention, regimen compliance, and programs of health behavior change. Building on models proposed by researchers in the areas of both family and individual stress, an integrated model is proposed for studying stress, illness, and health behavior. The *Multisystem Assessment of Stress and Health* (MASH) model is proposed, which offers a more comprehensive assessment of stress, coping resources and behaviors, and adaptation at four system levels: individual, family, marital, and work.

This chapter is based on a paper presented at the Applied Psychology Conference on Behavioral Health Assessment held at Kent State University on July 30, 1988. Work on this chapter was supported in part by the Agricultural Experiment Station, University of Minnesota, St. Paul, MN.

INDIVIDUAL HEALTH AND FAMILY HEALTH

In one of the earliest comprehensive reviews of the family's impact on health, Litman (1974) suggested that since the family constitutes the most important social context within which illness occurs and is resolved, it should serve as the primary unit in health and medical care. However, the issue of whether the individual or the family can or should be the unit of analysis has long been a subject of debate among family researchers.

In a paper addressing the issue of family health, the World Health Organization (WHO) suggested that the notion of family health as currently used is often ambiguous (World Health Organization, 1976). While there may be health (as measured by the presence or absence of disease) in individual family members, the concept of family health is fraught with some difficulties. Only individuals have diseases. Though a family group might have effective and functional or ineffective and dysfunctional processes, it is argued that family health should be restricted to the sum of the health status of individual members of a family. But the health of a family is more than the sum of its parts. Therefore, WHO proposed that *familial health* connote "*the relative functioning of the family as the primary social agent in the promotion of health and well-being*" (WHO, 1976, p. 17). And since the family is the basic unit of human social organization, it might very well be the most desired unit for preventive and therapeutic intervention.

In a similar vein, Turk and Kerns (1985) pointed out the need to consider the importance of the role of family on the maintenance of health and the response to illness across the life cycle. They suggested that studies in behavioral medicine and health psychology need to move away from the conventional medical model, with its focus upon the individual, and consider the major context in which illness occurs and in which health is maintained—namely, the family system.

The fields of behavioral medicine and health psychology have recently begun to give more attention to the characteristics of families and family systems at all phases of health and illness. Their efforts have benefited from the work of family sociologists and some social psychologists, whose efforts have resulted in more comprehensive family theories that can then be applied in the study of psychopathology within families, family stress, and family health behaviors. These family theorists and researchers have attempted to conceptualize and measure unique family system properties as opposed to individual properties within groups.

DIMENSIONS OF FAMILY SYSTEMS

Some of the earliest work in conceptualizing group properties within families was done by Angell (1936), who identified two dimensions of families: *family integration* and *family adaptability. Integration* was defined as the family's bonds of coherence, in terms of the common interests, affections, and economic interdependence. *Family adaptability* referred to the family's flexibility as a unit in meeting difficulties and the family's readiness to adjust to changed situations.

In Hill's (1949) study of families under stress, these two dimensions were used to understand war separation and reunion. He combined these two measures into a measure he referred to as *dynamic stability.* Later, the general systems theories of von Bertalanffy (1968) and Buckley (1967) had an important influence on family systems theory and family therapy.

A number of family theorists have, over the past 20 years, developed a wide range of descriptive variables that provides a comprehensive and realistic view of the family. These concepts have been subsumed under the three integrative dimensions of cohesion, adaptability, and communication by Olson (1986) in the development and refinement of the *Circumplex Model of Family Systems* (see Table 1).

The salience of *family cohesion, adaptability,* and *communication* is that various family theorists, researchers, and therapists have utilized concepts which can be subsumed under these three dimensions. Beavers and Voeller (1983) described two family forces, centripetal and centrifugal, which are similar to the notions of family integration and cohesion; family adaptability is the second dimension. Their system model focuses on increasing levels of growth from entropy (death of a system) to negentropy (system growth), seeing family adaptability as a linear dimension. Benjamin (1974, 1977) suggested concepts of affiliation and interdependence. Epstein, Bishop, and Bishop (1983) developed the McMaster Model of Family Functioning using concepts of affective involvement (similar to cohesion), behavior control and problem solving (similar to adaptability), and communication and affective responsiveness (communication). French and Guidera's (1974) concepts of power and the capacity to change are similar to adaptability. Gottman's (1979) concepts of validation and contrasting also parallel cohesion and adaptability.

One of the typologies developed include Kantor and Lehr's (1975) open, closed, and random systems. Family members play four basic parts: the mover, follower, opposer, and bystander. The dimensional goals were affect, power, and meaning. Focusing on family functioning in studies of both clinical and nonclinical families, L'Abate (1985) proposed the concepts of intimacy and power. Leary (1957) and Constantine (1977) proposed concepts of affection–hostility and dominance–submission, which parallel cohesion and adaptability.

Leff and Vaughan (1985) suggested the concepts of distance and problem-solving, while Lewis, Beavers, Gossett, and Phillips (1977) proposed the concepts of closeness and power. Parsons and Bales (1955) proposed the expressive and instrumental roles within families, which are similar to the concepts of cohesion and adaptability. Finally, the intensive experimental studies of Reiss

TABLE 1 Theoretical models of family systems utilizing concepts related to cohesion, adaptability, and communication dimensions

Researcher(s)	Cohesion	Adaptability	Communication	Others
Beavers and Voeller (1983)	Centripetal (systemic growth) Centrifugal	Adaptability	Affect	
Benjamin (1974, 1977)	Affiliation	Interdependence		
Epstein, Bishop, and Levin (1978)	Affective involvement	Behavior control Problem solving Roles	Communication Affective responsiveness	
French and Guidera (1974)		Capacity to change Power		Anxiety Role as symptom carrier
Gottman (1979)	Validation	Contrasting		
Kantor and Lehr (1975)	Affect	Power		Meaning
L'Abate (1985)	Intimacy	Power		
Leary (1957) and Constantine (1977)	Affection–hostility	Dominance–submission		
Leff and Vaughn (1985)	Distance	Problem solving		
Lewis, Beavers, Gossett, and Phillips (1976)	Closeness	Power	Affect	Mythology
Parsons and Bales (1955)	Expressive role	Instrumental role		
Reiss (1981)	Coordination	Closure		

(1981) relied heavily on a paradigm focusing on family problem-solving employing the dimensions of coordination (similar to cohesion) and closure (similar to the concept of change or adaptability).

FAMILY ASSESSMENT: BRIDGING THE GAP BETWEEN THEORY AND RESEARCH

In the past, advancement in the field of family theory and family research has been retarded by a lack of effective assessment instruments. In an attempt to bridge this gap between these family theories, family research, and practice, a variety of self-report family assessment instruments have been developed (Cromwell, Olson, & Fournier, 1976; Cromwell & Peterson, 1983; Olson, 1986).

Four family inventories selected for a review by Olson (1987) met the following criteria: (1) they tapped the relevant theoretical dimensions mentioned above and (2) they are highly developed psychometrically, with continued attempts made to improve their reliability, validity, and clinical utility. The four inventories are the *Family Environmental Scale* (FES) developed by Moos (1974), the *Family Assessment Device* (FAD) constructed by Epstein and colleagues (1983), the *Family Assessment Measure* (FAM III) developed by Skinner, Steinauer, and Santa Barbara (1983), and the *Family Adaptability and Cohesion Evaluation Scales* (FACES III) developed by Olson, Portner, and Lavee (1985).

Table 2 indicates the theoretical dimensions of cohesion, adaptability, and communication and how the specific scales in each of these four instruments relate to these three dimensions. In the *Family Environmental Scale* (FES), the cohesion and independence scale relates to the cohesion dimension; the control and organizational scales relate to adaptability; and the expressiveness and conflict scales relate to the communication dimension. There are also four scales that do not fit into these categories: the achievement orientation, active–recreational orientation, intellectual–cultural orientation, and the moral–religious emphasis scales.

The *Family Assessment Device* (FAD) has an affective involvement scale that assesses cohesion; while behavior control, problem-solving, and roles assess the communication dimension. The *Family Assessment Measure* (FAM III) has concepts and scales similar to the FAD scales. Affective involvement taps the cohesion dimension; task performance, role performance, and control tap the adaptability dimension; and communication and affective expression relate to the communication dimension. Values and norms is the only category that does not seem to fit into the three dimensions.

Finally, the *Family Adaptability and Cohesion Evaluation Scales* (FACES III) assess the cohesion and adaptability dimensions. Separate scales have been developed to assess ENRICH marital communication (Olson, Fournier, &

TABLE 2 Four family inventories related to major family dimensions

Inventory	Cohesion	Adaptability	Communication	Other
Family Environment Scale (FES)	Cohesion Independence	Organization Control	Expressiveness Conflict	Achievement Active–recreational Moral–religious Intellectual–cultural
Family Assessment Device (FAD)	Affective involvement	Problem solving Behavior control Roles	Communication Affective responsiveness	Responsiveness
Family Norms Measure (FAM III)	Affective involvement	Task accomplishment Control Role performance	Communication Affective expression	Values and norms
Family Adaptability & Cohesion Evaluation Scales (FACES III)	Cohesion	Adaptability	Marital communication Parent–adolescent communication	

Druckman, 1986) and parent–adolescent communication (Barnes & Olson, 1985).

FAMILY VARIABLES AND FAMILY HEALTH BEHAVIOR

Comprehensive Overview by Campbell

These family measures and others have proven useful for investigators in studying the interaction of family functioning and the health of individual family members. In a comprehensive review of the family's impact on health, Campbell (1986) addresses both conceptual and methodological issues in examining the family's impact on both physical and mental health. Adapting a rating system used by Sackett and Haynes (1976) to rate compliance studies, Campbell examined the research design, selection of subjects, the family (independent) variable, and the illness or outcome (dependent) variable. Without reference to specific studies, Table 3 briefly summarizes his review of various studies that examine the family's influence on physical and mental health.

Among the family variables represented in the studies in Campbell's review were demographic and structural characteristics, such as marital status, age of family members, number of children, ethnic background, and socioeconomic status. More dynamic family variables included stressful life events, family interaction, and family functioning.

Some conclusions that Campbell offers from these studies are that a range of family variables such as marital status and support, family involvement, family conflict and poor organization, and family support play important roles in CHD, hypertension, diabetic control, and compliance. Likewise, parental communication deviance, expressed emotion, critical comments by relatives, family interactions, rigid interactions, and distant fathers and overinvolved mothers have been major factors in understanding schizophrenia, depression, alcoholism and drug abuse, and anorexia.

Studies examining the impact of the family on health and health behavior will be reviewed in greater detail below. Emphasis will be upon those studies that have attempted to utilize a systems framework in their investigations of primary prevention behaviors, hypertension, regimen compliance, health beliefs, and health behavior changes programs (see summary of studies in Table 4).

Pratt's Energized Family

Some of the earliest research examining the impact of the family system on the family's health and health behavior was done by Lois Pratt in her work on the "energized family" (Pratt, 1976). Pratt's thesis was that energized families

TABLE 3 Summary of studies on the family's impact on physical and mental health

Health problem	Family variables	Results
Physical health		
Overall mortality	Death of spouse	Substantial evidence shows increase in mortality of men after death of spouse
	Social support (marital status, no. of contacts with relatives, no. of living children)	Social ties and supports have a major influence on overall mortality, and the family is the most important element of support
Cardiovascular heart disease	Marital status, spousal support, family environment, family support, family problems, spouse's attitude, marital dissatisfaction, divorce	Family factors, especially spousal support, affect mortality due to hypertension after myocardial infarction, and family factors influence hypertension with increased compliance with medication and weight control; weak evidence to show the family affecting the development of heart disease
Diabetes	Family environment, family functioning, family type, parent behaviors	Correlations have been found between poor family functioning and diabetic control; diabetic families tend to be more rigid than most families, but evidence for enmeshment is contradictory; family stress could have direct physiological effect on a child's diabetes
Asthma	Family education, family situation, family therapy, removal of family	Family therapy is effective in treatment of asthma; family education is associated with better management, less fear
Various childhood illnesses	Stressful family life events, chronic family stress	Stressful events are associated with duration but not number of infections; high stress is associated with certain complications; 30% of strep infections are preceded by family stress
Pregnancy complications	Stress, family support, psychologial assets	High stress and low tangible social supports are associated with certain complications; women with high stress are protected from complications by psychosocial assets
Obesity	Spouse/mother involvement, spouse reinforcement	Spouse involvement is positively associated with maintaining weight loss; separating mother and child in treatment was most helpful

TABLE 3 Summary of studies on the family's impact on physical and mental health (*Continued*)

Health problem	Family variables	Results
Physical health		
Smoking	Partner support	Partner helpfulness predicted smoking cessation
Mental health		
Schizophrenia	Parental communication deviance	High parental communication deviance has been found to be present before development of symptoms; both genetic and familial variables influence the development of schizophrenia
Depression	Family environment, mental health of biological parents/spouse, perceived parental care, marital disputes, family and childhood history	The presence of a depressed parent and style of parental rearing may influence the development of depression in later years; a decrease in marital disputes is correlated with a decrease of depressive symptoms; depressed patients scored parents as less caring and more controlling; children of depressed parents had more psychopathology
Alcoholism	Marital interaction, family participation, marital conflict resolution, alcoholism in family	Family involvement is associated with completion of treatment
	Communication style, marital satisfaction, family stress and functioning, role functioning congruence	Decreased drinking is associated with fewer symptoms in spouse but not patient; relapsed families had less cohesion, expressiveness, and congruence than recovered families
Drug abuse	Intrafamily perceptions, mother–child symbiosis, family life, family environment and interactions, family hierarchy	Addicts and parents describe addicts as passive, dependent; mothers of addicts scored high in symbiosis; family conflict and lack of initimacy are associated with heroin use; addicts perceive parents as having high achievement orientation, low conflict; more hierarchical reversals and cross-generational conflicts were associated with addiction
Anorexia nervosa	Family characteristics	Lack of leadership, covert coalitions, self-sacrifice, facade of unity, rigidity, and lack of conflict resolution were associated with anorexia in the family

Note. From Campbell (1986). Adapted by permission.

TABLE 4 Family dimensions and health behaviors

Study	Family dimensions	Health
Pratt's "Energized Family"		
Pratt (1976)	Freedom and responsiveness, interaction, role structure, coping effort, links to community	Health problems
Primary prevention behaviors: Obesity studies		
Hartz et al. (1977)	Family environment	Obesity among children
Khoury et al. (1983)	Family environment	Body mass of parents to children
Ashton (1983)	Family-influenced exercise	Activity of parents to children
Perrier (1979)	Parental attitudes and interests	Active versus nonactive children
Kleges et al. (in press)	Family interaction patterns	Obesity among children
Hypertension and interaction patterns within the family		
Diamond (1982)	Unexpressed anger/hostility	Hypertension
Baer et al. (1980) Baer et al. (1983)	Interaction patterns during conflict, eye contact of fathers during conflict	Hypertension in fathers Hypertension in fathers
Julius et al. (1987)	Anger expressed/held in, level of guild, leaving/staying during conflict	Hypertension, mortality rates
Regimen compliance		
Glasgow, McCaul, and Dreher (1983)	Family discord and positive family functioning	Compliance with diabetic regimens in children
Gath, Smith, and Baum (1980)	Family conflict	Control of diabetic children
Simonds (1977)	Divorce rate	Control of diabetes
Steidl et al. (1980)	Efficiency of problem solving, coalitions and boundaries, openness to opinions and feelings, sharing of power in marriage, personal responsibility	Compliance with hemodialysis
Doherty et al. (1983)	Spousal support	Health belief and compliance with cholesterol lowering medication

TABLE 4 Family dimensions and health behaviors (*Continued*)

Study	Family dimensions	Health
Health beliefs		
Charney et al. (1967) Becker et al. (1972, 1974) Francis et al. (1969)	Mother's perception of severity of illness	Giving medication to child
Elling et al. (1960)	Mother's belief in efficacy	Administration of penicillin, other medicines; keeping clinic appointments
Becker et al. (1972)	Concern with role of "good mother"	Compliance, seeking of medical care versus self-treatment
Heinzelmann and Bagley (1970)	Spousel influence: desire to please	Beginning and continuing exercise program
Goldsen, Gerhardt, and Candy (1957) King and Leach (1951)	Defensive generalizations in the family	Delay in seeking care
Health behavior change programs		
Wilson and Brownell (1978) Brownell et al. (1978)	Stopping criticism of wife, giving positive reinforcement	Success in weight control program for obese women
Pearce, LeBow, and Orchard (1981)	Stopping nagging of spouse	Losing weight and maintaining loss
Brownell, Kelman, and Stunkard (1983)	Level of involvement between parent and adolescent	Weight loss
Nader et al. (1983)	Offering of social support	Changing diet and exercise patterns

have more positive health behaviors. This energized family as conceptualized by Pratt is very similar in its functioning to Olson's notion of the "balanced" family on the Circumplex Model, that is, families that are balanced on dimensions of cohesion, adaptability, and communication; function more adequately; have more resources; and more adequately cope with stress (Olson, Russell, & Sprenkle, 1983; Olson, Sprenkle, & Russell, 1979).

Mechanic (1979) has argued that persons who may engage in one type of preventive behavior, such as a dietary change, may not necessarily change behavior in another area, such as seat belts. There is no "preventive personality" per se, and each behavioral pattern should be analyzed separately. However, Pratt has suggested that the energized family may be the type of family that might indeed be more likely to engage in a wide variety of preventive health behaviors. She hypothesized that members of the energized family

- interact with one another on a regular basis both inside and outside the home, in task and leisure activities and through general conversation;
- have regular contact with groups and organizations outside the family, such as medical, educational, political, recreational, and business groups;
- attempt to master their lives by taking responsibility for themselves and seeking out information to improve their diet or exercise patterns;
- employ a fluid internal role organization where roles are flexible, power is shared, decision-making is shared, and members are supportive of the personal growth of other members;
- have freedom to explore healthy development; and
- have an energy that comes from regular interaction between the persons inside the family and persons or groups outside the family.

Pratt conducted a study of 273 families to test the hypothesis that energized families will have better health than members of nonenergized families. There were five dimensions of family structure that she correlated with the extent of health promotions of men, women, children, and the combined family. These were (a) freedom and responsiveness, (b) interaction, (c) role structure, (d) coping effort, and (e) links to the community.

It was found that in the freedom and responsiveness dimension, a high level of aversive control of the child by the parents was significantly related to a high level of health problems among the children and also the men and women. This is the kind of punishment that tends to control and restrain the child by aversive means, such as physical force, withdrawing privileges, verbal abuse, hostile reaction, or ridicule.

On the contrary, a high level of automony for the child, or the level of responsibility given the child plus the opportunity given the child to develop his or her uniqueness, was significantly associated with a low level of health problems in women and children and the combined family. In this same direction, a high level of obstructive conflict between the husband and wife was significantly related to extensive health problems among all family members. This is the type of conflict in which the husband or wife might block each other's efforts to function by physical force, physical separation, noncooperation, or nonperformance in such areas as finances, preparing meals, and sexual relations.

In the interaction among family members dimension, it was found that a high level of interaction among members was associated with fewer health problems, but the relationships were not consistent or very strong. In the coping dimension, parents training of children in health matters was significantly correlated with fewer health problems for women, but not for men and children. Pratt did not see this dimension as a major influence on health. In the conjugal role structure dimension, a flexible division of labor in the care of the children's health was significantly related to lower health problems for men, but not for women and children. Also, conjugal power was not found to be a significant factor in the level of health problems of the men, women, or children. In the family's links to the community dimension, it was found that the participation of family members in community organizations was not significantly related to the health of family members. There was one significant exception. When the overall level of community participation by the whole family was high, women had much better health or fewer health problems than when the family group had a generally lower level of community participation.

The stepwise regression analysis revealed that punishment, obstructive conflict, autonomy, support for the child, and (somewhat less so) interaction among family members were the most influential aspects of family structure for the health of family members. After these measures of family structures were taken into account in the regression analysis, the dimensions of conjugal role structure and community participation were found to have no additional influence.

A stepwise regression was done to examine the combined influence of these significant dimensions of family structure. It was found that these dimensions accounted for 16% of the variance in health problems for men, 25% of the variance in health problems for women, and 27% of the variance in health problems for children.

Pratt (1976) concluded that it is the family's overall pattern and not separate characteristics that affects the health of family members. Thus, the climate of health and the patterns of interaction and organization within the family have a strong and independent influence on the health of individual family members.

The Family and Primary Prevention Behaviors

Baranowski and Nader (1985) point out that no other studies have been reported that verify Pratt's findings. There are, however, a number of other studies in primary prevention literature that address various aspects of health behaviors and family structure or family functioning. Hartz, Giefer, and Rimm (1977) studied over 73,000 members of TOPS (Take Off Pounds Sensibly) and found that from 32% to 39% of the variation in obesity among children was due to variables related to the family environment, while only 11% was due to genetic factors. Khoury, Morrison, Laskarzewski, and Glueck (1983) studied the relationships between body mass of parents and children and found that the immediate family environment was the crucial component in predicting body mass of the children living at home, but not the adult children living away from home.

Exercise as a preventive health behavior also has been shown to come under the influence of the family. Ashton (1983) indicated that the physical activity of parents, especially those of the mother, correlated with the activity patterns of the children. In a national sample survey, the Perrier Corporation (1979) found that parental attitudes and interests in sports discriminated between active and nonactive children. Waxman and Stunkard (1980), in an observational study of obese and nonobese children, found that in the homes of the obese children there was much less activity by the children than in the homes of the nonobese children. Seventy-four percent of the obese children spent time sitting, while only 49% of the nonobese children spent time in this way. Kleges and others (in press) found similar results in an observational study of activity and family interaction patterns of families with young children. They developed and validated an observational protocol for observing and recording the activity and simultaneous family interaction patterns of young children in these families. During the 90 minutes after the "typical" family dinner, the authors found that an obese child was significantly less active than a nonobese child. Also, the nonobese child received three times as many encouragements to be active as the obese child.

Baranowski and Nader (1985) point out that although most studies on families and exercise suggest exercise as protective of heart disease, accurate methods of assessing aerobic activity need to be developed and validated. Although there have been studies showing strong support for the role of families in affecting the activity levels of their children, no literature has been found on husband-wife exercise patterns or how behaviors of husbands or wives affect their spouse's activity level.

The Family and Hypertension

Studies on hypertension and interaction patterns within the family have revealed significant results regarding family behavior and family health outcomes. Specifically, they have shown that unexpected anger and hostility in the family can lead to hypertension (Diamond, 1982). Baer, Vincent, Williams, Bourianoff, and Bartlett (1980) set up an exercise for families with hypertensive fathers and families with nonhypertensive fathers, the mothers and children in both families being nonhypertensive. Both sets of families were given a conflict-laden task to perform and the interactions were recorded on videotape and analyzed for verbal and nonverbal behavior. It was found that when families with hypertensive fathers were given the conflict-laden tasks to perform, the fathers in these families produced more negative behavior or behavior that reflected hostility or interpersonal rejection.

In a replication of these studies, Baer and others (1983) found that these hypertensive fathers were more likely not to look at another family member when talking. That is, he would avert his gaze from the mother and children. This averted gaze was more likely to occur during periods of conflict or negative verbalizations than during periods of nonconflict. This was interpreted to suggest that families with hypertensive fathers were more likely to avoid conflict than confront and resolve the conflict. These patterns of conflict avoidance lead to suppression of anger and hostility, which in turn has been shown to be related to high blood pressure.

Julius, Harburg, Cottington, and Johnson (1987) examined prospectively (1971–1983) the relationship between anger-coping types, blood pressure, and all-cause mortality in a sample of men and women ages 30 to 69 years (n = 696). The anger types were keeping anger in or letting anger out. These anger-coping types were assessed by self-report of subjects to two hypothetical anger-provoking situations involving an unjustified attack by a power figure. In one instance the person was a policeman; in the other scenario, it was one's spouse or sweetheart. Participants were asked to "imagine that your (husband/wife/sweetheart) yelled in anger or blew up at you for something that wasn't your fault." For each situation, three factors were measured: (a) whether anger would be expressed or not, (b) the level of guilt that would result if there was a display of anger, and (c) whether or not the subject would leave or stay and protest the unprovoked attack.

While the hypothesis that suppressed anger would be directly related to higher blood pressure was not supported, an item analysis of the anger–coping items revealed that two out of three anger-coping items measuring a response to an unjustified attack by one's spouse did predict mortality risk. Individuals who held their anger in were 2.4 times as likely to die over the follow-up period than those who would express their anger. This was significant at the $p > .001$ level. In addition, those respondents who did not protest an unjustified attack by their spouse were 1.7 times as likely to have died during the follow-up period compared with those who protested the attack ($p = .023$).

Comparing indices of suppressed anger, individuals who scored high on suppressed anger (that is, they held their anger in, felt guilty, and did not protest the unjustified attack) were 2.1 times as likely to have died during the follow-up period as compared with those who scored low in suppressing anger (that is, they expressed their anger, did not feel guilty, and protested the unjustified attack). She concludes by stating that if the response to an angry attack is suppressed anger, if this response is consistent across many social situations, and the attacks are chronic (as they could be from a spouse), then a state of resentment will arise. In this state of resentment, the angry feelings and their biological processes are aroused by internal hostile attitudes as a chronic condition. Then, when this psychophysiological process of coping with anger interacts with elevated blood pressure, a morbid condition and mortality may result.

Clearly then, family rules about how anger can be expressed within the family system can have a significant impact on the health of individual family members. If the family rules permit a healthy expression of anger toward one's spouse, then the chances for better health outcomes can be increased. While not directly supporting Pratt's findings, Julius' study does seem to indicate that the pattern of conflict and communication within the family can play a significant role in the health of family members.

Pratt (1976) also suggested that the extent and variety of interactions within the family can be associated with fewer health problems. But while the extent and variety of interactions may be important within the family, and the family rules (patterns of emotional expression) about anger have important health consequences, as seen in the Julius study, so too family rules about what one is permitted to talk about can play a significant role in the health behaviors in families. For instance, how one can talk about fears of getting sick or fears of death from a potentially lethal disease such as cancer can have important long-term consequences, especially in the prediagnostic phase of an illness.

The Family and Regimen Compliance

The literature on regimen compliance provides insights into the role that family functioning and various family processes play in maintaining an effective level of health behavior in families. Baranowski and Nader (1985) suggest that, in general, there has been less of a relationship between regimen compliance and family structure (such as single versus dual parent household, number of children, education of parents or employment of head of household) than for family processes such as family cohesiveness or interference of regimen with social role tasks. Since regimen compliance has a highly decisional aspect to it, it is more likely to be influenced by family process variables than by family structure variables. However, as the medical problem becomes more severe, then even family structure variables will play a major role. For instance, since the procedures may be overwhelming financially, emotionally, and procedurally, having an absent father would significantly affect any compliance with kidney transplantation regimens.

In a study by Gath, Smith, and Baum (1980), this same pattern of family conflict and adversity was positively related to poorly controlled diabetic children. On the other side of this coin, Simonds (1977) found an unusually low rate of divorce in families of well-controlled patients, compared with groups with unstable diabetes or nondiabetic comparison groups.

The literature on adult compliance shows a similar pattern between family functioning and compliance. In a study by Steidl and others (1980) of 23 chronic hemodialysis patients, it was found that six of ten ratings of family functioning were significantly correlated with overall compliance. Those who complied were more likely to come from families who efficiently solved their problems, had strong coalitions between parents instead of any crossgenerational coalitions, had clear parent–child boundaries, were open and responsive to the opinions and feelings of others, had a marriage in which power was shared and negotiated differences, and had family members who assumed responsibility for their actions. It should be noted that the above characteristics are very similar to the characteristics of the balanced family on Olson's Circumplex Model. It is these families that Olson hypothesized will function more adequately under stress and across the life cycle (Olson et al., 1983).

A study by Doherty, Schrott, Metcalf, and Iasiello-Vailas (1983) examined the relationship between spousal support and health belief, and compliance with taking cholesterol lowering medication. Wives (n = 144) of middle-aged men who were participating in the Coronary Primary Prevention trial were the subjects. Compliance was measured by packet counts of unused medication (or placebo). Structured interviews were conducted with the wives, husbands, and medical staff to determine the kind and extent of the wives' support. There were also separate interviews with the wives to determine their health beliefs.

The results showed that all three measures of spousal support were highly correlated with compliance. Those subjects in the group with the highest spousal support averaged 96% compliance, while those in the lowest support group showed 70% compliance. The specific wife behaviors that were correlated with compliance were "showing an interest in the program" and "reminding him about his medicine or diet." However, "nagging him about his medicine or diet" was found to be negatively correlated with compliance. In addition, the health beliefs of the wife regarding the husband's susceptibility to the risks of elevated cholesterol and the benefits of treatment were found to be correlated with her self-report of her support of the husband.

Baranowski and Nader (1985) suggest directions for further research in this area by presenting the series of models shown in Figure 1. Model A indicates that the current thinking that can be inferred from the literature is that family functioning affects compliance, which then affects disease control. However, it might just as likely be possible that family functioning directly affects disease control, such as through emotional or stress-related mediating variables. Then family functioning affects compliance as well, as shown in Model B. Since many studies deal with cases of chronic degenerative diseases, another possibility (Model C) for explaining the documented cross-sectional correlations is that poor disease control leads to additional problems to be faced by the family, which in turn leads to poorer family functioning and reduced compliance. Poor disease control may require more difficult regimens and pose other emotional problems for family functioning, and the compliance may cause problems in family functioning, which in turn exacerbate problems of disease control (Model D).

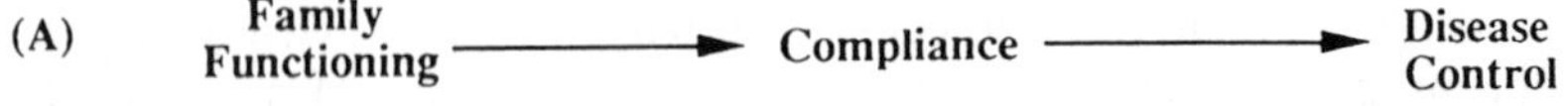

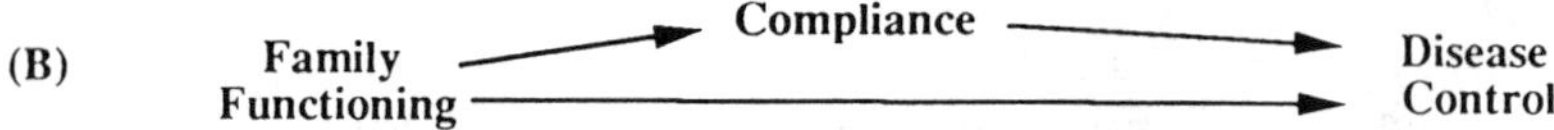

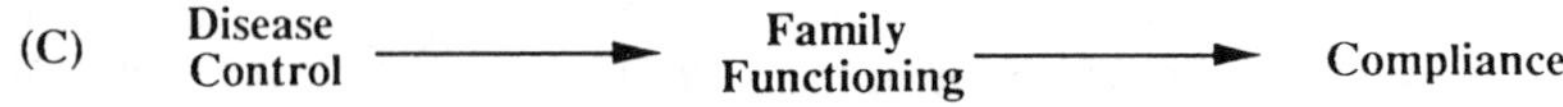

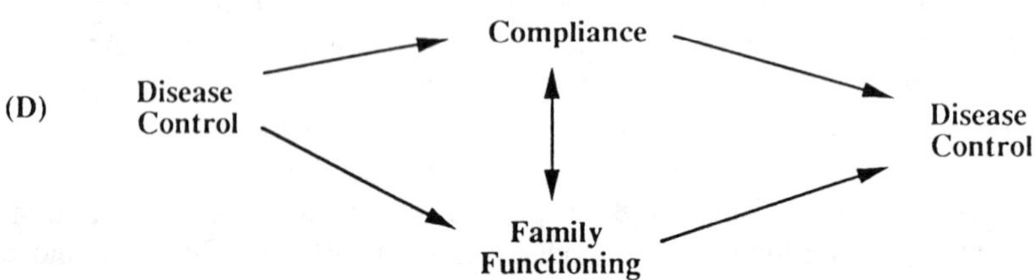

FIGURE 1 Models of family functioning, compliance, and disease control relationships. From "Family health behavior" by T. Baranowski and P. Nader. In *Health, Illness and Families,* D. Turk and R. D. Kerns (Eds.), 1985. New York: John Wiley & Sons. Copyright 1985. Used by permission.

Family Compliance and Health Beliefs

In reviewing the literature on families and compliance behavior, Becker and Green (1975) suggested that the health belief model can provide a framework for understanding the variables involved in promoting compliance within families. This model suggests that the person's subjective perception of his or her relative susceptibility to the particular health condition, his or her perception of the problem severity (organically and socially) of the consequences of contracting the disease, and the individual's evaluation of how helpful (the potential benefits) he or she believes his behavior will be weighed against the perception of physical, psychological, or financial barriers to taking such action.

In support of this framework, Charney and others (1967) found, in research conducted in several pediatric practices, that the mother's perception of the severity of the disease at the onset was significantly related to the likelihood of giving the medication. Other studies have found similar associations between the perceived seriousness of the illness (both in terms of organic severity and interference with the mother's activities) and compliance with medication therapy and keeping of appointments (Becker, Drachman, & Kirscht, 1972, 1974; Francis, Korsch, & Morris, 1969).

In keeping with this health belief model, Elling, Whittemore, and Green (1960) also found that the mother's belief in the efficacy of clinical medication could predict regular administrations of penicillin, and her belief in the doctor's ability to cure illness was related to how faithful she was in keeping clinic appointments. Furthermore, Becker and others (1972) found that compliant mothers worried more about being a "good mother" and were more concerned about health matters in general than were noncompliant mothers. These compliant mothers would more likely seek medical treatment when symptoms arose in their children than try some form of self-treatment.

Again, the nature of the family processes as well as the level of family cohesiveness can be a major factor in compliance, as demonstrated in a study by Heinzelmann and Bagley (1970) which examined the influence that the spouse played in undertaking and continuing a fitness exercise program related to coronary heart disease. At the beginning of the program, the volunteers rated the "desire to please their wives" as lowest of their motivations to undertake the fitness exercise program. However in subsequent analyses it was found that of those men whose wives' attitudes toward the program were positive, 80% had good or excellent patterns of compliance. For those whose wives had neutral or negative attitudes toward the exercise program, only 40% had good or excellent patterns of adherence.

The marital relationship can play a major role in patterns of regimen compliance. Spousal attitude can be a significant factor in how well one participates in behaviors that will prevent one from becoming sick, and will lead to improved health as well.

A number of studies have also examined the impact that various beliefs held by the family has in the prediagnostic phase of illness. Leventhal, Leventhal, and Nguyen (1985) suggest that the severity of the impact of illness in adult members varies with a number of factors: (a) the biological type of illness (e.g., cancer, cardiovascular disease); (b) the stage of the illness (i.e., prediagnostic, diagnostic and treatment, rehabilitation and control, or recurrence); (c) the structure of the family; (d) the identity of the sick person (e.g., mother, father, grandparent); (e) the point in the person's life span that the illness occurs; and (f) the point in the life course of the family and culture at which the illness occurs.

Some researchers have suggested that the family may play a significant role in increasing the delay in seeking care for the illness (Goldson, Gerhardt, & Handy, 1957; King & Leach, 1951). This might be because the family encourages denial of the feelings of vulnerability associated with a potentially lethal disease, such as cancer. Such defensiveness and denial by the family may lead to inaccurate identification of early warning signs of the illness (Leventhal et al., 1985). Closed communication such as this could prove to be potentially very harmful to the health of individual family members.

One of Pratt's dimensions of the family system was the extent and variety of interaction among members. While her study suggested that there was not a very strong or consistent association between such open and varied communication and fewer family health problems (Pratt, 1976), other studies seem to indicate that a significant association might indeed exist in some families.

Such mismatches between the perceived threat, due to various psychological defenses, and the actual pathophysiological course of the disease can lead to a failure to delay the onset or to control the spread of a chronic disease (Leventhal et al., 1985). Fatalistic attitudes that people have toward some chronic diseases could lead to a failure to respond in enough time to control the disease. Dent and Goulston (1982) found that one third to one half of the respondents in a random survey of 500 adults were either uncertain or agreed that cancer was preventable. And an even slightly higher percentage of respondents believed that cancer could not be controlled once it is contracted.

While it may be that the perceived threat of an illness affects family functioning in such a way as to delay the taking of appropriate preventive action, the reverse might also be true. That is, the level of family functioning, including the levels of adaptability, cohesion, and communication, might be such that the family cannot respond to perceive threats appropriately. The family system might be too chaotic or too disengaged, or communication might be so incomplete that a family might find itself unable to respond effectively to the impending crisis.

The Family and Health Behavior Change Programs

While the literature on families and compliance behavior reveals the influence of the family system on response to specific required medical regimens, the literature on how families respond to health behavior change programs can also shed light on the impact that family structure and family interaction have upon health within the family. The studies on compliance were naturalistic in that they studied how families respond to required medical regimens with no attempt to manipulate or directly influence change within the family. The following studies were programs that were designed to change either various health behaviors within the family or regimen compliance behavior. This was done by either systematically varying family involvement as a controlled experimental variable or studying the family as a whole as the unit of intervention.

One of the first experimental studies of couple involvement in weight loss programs was done by Wilson and Brownell (1978). They found no effect of involving or not involving husbands of obese women in a behavioral program for weight loss. The husbands attended eight training sessions in which they were taught various behavior modification principles that included being instructed to stop criticizing their partners' weight and eating behaviors, and being trained to give positive reinforcement when appropriate and to help their wives arrange the conditions and consequences of eating at home.

However, in a follow-up study, Brownell, Heckerman, Westlake, Hayes, and Monti (1978) assigned 29 obese men and women to one of two conditions: couple training as in the previous experiment, or subjects alone without their spouses. Then they created a third category of noncooperative spouses, in which persons whose spouses refused to participate were assigned to a third group. Immediately after the 10-session intervention, no statistically significant differences were found across the three groups; but at the 3- and 6-month follow-ups, there were statistically significant differences in the couple-training group versus the other two groups.

In a study by Pearce, LeBow, and Orchard (1981), the best results for losing weight and keeping it off were obtained when the nonparticipating spouse was asked to not nag or otherwise give the spouse a hard time in regard to the weight loss. Thus, removing the spouse as a detriment to change proved to be just as important as training the spouse to be helpful. This would seem to be consistent with Pratt's (1976) findings regarding the role that "obstructive conflict" plays in family health.

In a study on the influence of parent–child intervention on weight loss by adolescents, Brownell, Kelman, and Stunkard (1983) varied the level of involvement between parent and adolescent in a weight loss program. Subjects were trained in cognitive and behavioral techniques, with one group in which the parent and child were trained together, another group in which the parent and child were trained separately, and a third group in which the child was trained alone. The results indicated that adolescents in the group where parents and children were trained separately achieved the greatest posttreatment weight loss. In addition, they were the only group to sustain the weight loss at a 1-year follow-up.

Brownell and his associates interpreted these results to indicate that the difference in adolescent weight loss across groups was due to the moderate level of involvement of the parents. The groups in which the parents were disengaged or overinvolved either gave the child too much freedom or exacerbated the usual parent–adolescent conflicts.

However, many of these studies are difficult to compare, since the participants vary on a variety of important characteristics. Some studies have used obese women alone, others have used men and women. Many of the studies do not provide an adequate discrimination in background variables such as ethnicity, employment status, or social class. In addition, the number of intervention sessions have varied from 6 to 18 sessions, and the extent of the interventions has varied greatly in both content and intensity. Further, many of the studies have ignored family systems theory and have involved spouses or significant others in an ad hoc fashion. These same criticisms could also be made of many of the studies in the cardiovascular-risk-reduction literature. Therefore, because of this lack of consistency it has been difficult to make useful interpretations of these results (Baranowski & Nader, 1985).

The various interpersonal mechanisms that families employ to be useful to one another in any health behavior change program has not always been made very clear. Social support, however, generally has been shown to be a key factor in success of various programs. In a study examining social support in a program to change diet and exercise patterns within families, the investigators found that social support was not offered very frequently at the beginning of the program, but that is increased at the end of the program in the experimental group over the control group (Nader, Baranowski, Vanderpool, Dworkin, & Dunn, 1983).

In a Gallup survey commissioned by *American Health* magazine (June 1985), it was found that families play a significant role in health behavior. Gallup interviewed 1,011 adults, asking them how they changed and who helped them change. They found that a spouse or significant other is more likely to influence a person's health habits than anyone else, including the family doctor. Husbands were twice as likely, for instance, to quit smoking (22% vs. 11%) and more likely to lose weight (42% vs. 31%) than single men. In general, they found that people who are separated, widowed, or divorced do less for their health than the married or the still-single (*American Health,* October 1985).

FAMILY STRESS AND ADAPTATION

In early stress research on the family, the outcome was the degree of crisis in the family social system following the stressor event (Hill, 1949, 1958). In the crisis situation, old patterns of family interaction and problem-solving were found to be inadequate and new patterns were needed. Stress was assessed by the degree to which the family system became disrupted and incapacitated and could not restore stability. However, Hanson and Johnson (1979) argued that such disruptions are not always unwelcome, nor do they always result in negative consequences for the family. Sometimes the family might even welcome the changes and see them as opportunities to restructure in a more positive manner.

This is congruent with systems theorists who suggest that living systems tend to evolve toward greater complexity (von Bertalanffy, 1968).

McCubbin and Patterson (1983) suggested that a continuum of adaptation might be a more useful concept to describe the postcrisis adjustment of the family. They propose a Double ABCX model of stress adaptation, building on the earliest work of Hill and Hanson (Hill, 1949, 1958; Hanson & Hill, 1964). They took Hill and Hanson's ABCX model and added postcrisis variables to move from an outcome of crisis to one of a continuum of adaptation. The focus in this model is on the postcrisis situation and the additional life stressors and strains that affect the family's adaptation, intrafamily and social resources used, any changes in the definition and meaning that the family makes to move out of the post-crisis situation, and a range of adaptational outcomes (see Figure 2).

In the Double ABCX Model, Hill's A Factor is seen as an accumulation or pile-up of stressors to produce the aA Factor. This pile-up of stressors or demands may come from the initial stressor and its demands and also subsequent hardships, normative transitions, prior strains, the consequences of the family efforts to cope, and ambiguity.

Hill's B Factor is the family's crisis-meeting resources in individual family members, the family unit, and in the community. This includes existing resources and resources that are already part of the family's repertoire, such as role flexibility or togetherness and expanded resources. It also includes resources that are new, expanded, or developed (e.g., education, role responsibilities) and social support from kin, friends, extended family, the church and other places in the community.

Hill's C Factor in the Double ABCX Model (the cC Factor) is the family's efforts to give meaning to the initial stressor, as well as additional stressors that follow in its wake, and efforts to bring the family back into balance. This involves clarifying issues to make them more manageable, decreasing the emotional intensity of the crisis situation, and giving encouragement to one another as everyone goes on with the business of being a family. The difference between the C and cC Factors relates to the general orientation to the overall situation in which the family has found itself. In the X Factor, the amount of crisis that results in the family system is a major outcome variable referring to disruptions in family routines in the wake of a family stress. The Double ABCX Model (the xX Factor) includes the three elements of the individual, the family system, and the community in which the family resides. Adaptation involves achieving a demand-capability balance between the individual and family, and between the family and community, and achieving a sense of coherence. Nonadaptation occurs when a balance is achieved on the individual–family–community levels. Maladaptation results when there is imbalance at the individual or family level, resulting in deterioration of family integrity, personal health, or loss of family independence.

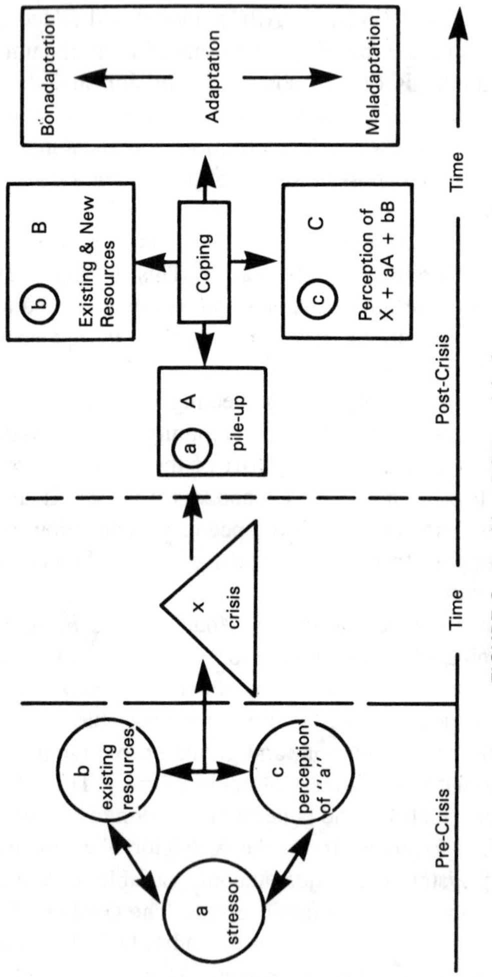

FIGURE 2 Double ABCX model of stress.

This progression from pathogenic models, which have illness or psychopathology as an outcome, to salutogenic models, which have wellness as an outcome, has been suggested by Antonovsky (1987) as an important distinction for the field of stress research. He argues that we cannot assume that stressors are intrinsically bad. While some indeed might be, there are others that might be neutral, others that might even be salutary for the individual, and still others that might have both negative and positive outcomes for the individual.

The same might also be said for families. Lavee, McCubbin, and Olson (1987) found that family strains were positively associated with more positive appraisal of the stressful situation. When marital adjustment was held constant, family strain increased the sense of coherence (the general orientation that things will work out well) within the family. The experience of overcoming their difficulties may have a salutary effect on families by bolstering their sense of competence and confidence.

What is needed in stress research, according to Antonovsky, are more studies of those persons and families that do well, even prosper in the face of stress. Instead of studying the symptoms of disease, we might learn much by studying the symptoms of wellness. All of us are constantly being bombarded by stressors. As the study by Lavee, Olson, and McCubbin (1988) indicates, some family system types respond better to these ongoing stressors and strains than others. The heart of Antonovsky's salutogenic model involves the study of successful coping or behavioral immunology. Instead of studying what keeps people from getting sick, Antonovsky argues, we should ask ourselves what facilitates a person to get healthier? He suggests that coping variables need to be abstracted one step higher in order to find "generalized resistance resources" that will help researchers and scholars better understand how the individual copes successfully to reinforce health.

FAMILY SYSTEM TYPES AND FAMILY STRESS

This generalized resistance resource that Antonovsky refers to is similar to Hill's (1949) crisis proof family and Pratt's (1976) energized family. This raises an interesting question: Are there certain characteristics a family might possess, or certain ways of structuring its interactions, allocating its roles, and successfully dealing with its issues of cohesion and intimacy that will make its members more resilient in the face of crisis or more resistant to stressors or strains? That is, might certain levels of the system constructs of cohesion, adaptability, and communication act in such a way as to make a family less vulnerable to stress and illness or better able to cope with stressors and strains once they have occurred?

These family constructs have been studied in family stress research, yielding interesting and useful results. For example, in a recent study by Lavee and others (1987), families with different system types were examined in relation to normative and nonnormative stressor events. The purpose of the study was to examine the relations among the same variables–events, transitions, intrafamilial strain, marital adjustment, sense of coherence, and well-being for four family system types based on the Circumplex Model (Olson et al., 1979).

The Circumplex Model has the two orthogonal dimensions of cohesion (defined as the amount of emotional bonding in the system) and adaptability (defined as the degree the system changes its roles and rules) in a space–property dimension. There are four levels of cohesion: disengaged (low cohesion), separated, connected, and enmeshed (very high cohesion); and four levels of adaptability: rigid (very low adaptability), structured, flexible, and chaotic (very high adaptability) (see Figure 3).

These system types of nonclinical families in this study were either high or low in cohesion (''separated'' or ''connected'') and either high or low in adaptability (''structured'' or ''flexible''), thus being in the ''balanced'' area of the Circumplex Model.

Using the LISREL VI program, a structural equation model of family well-being following the pileup of stressful demands was analyzed using data from these four system types, holding the measurement model equal across the four types. The results revealed that in all four family system types, intrafamilial strain was intensified by recent changes—either stressful life events, normative transitions, or both. Also, in all family types, marital strength was related to intrafamilial strain and affected perceived coping resources of the family.

However, the effect of stressful life events on family functioning and well-being may be influenced by the family's system type. It was found that some effects in the stress model may be influenced primarily by family connectedness. For example, marital adjustment affects well-being, directly or indirectly, in ''connected'' but not in ''separated'' families. Other effects are accounted for primarily by family flexibility, for example, the direct effect of intrafamilial strain on well-being in ''flexible'' but not in ''structured'' families.

Furthermore, the results suggested that a combination of cohesion and flexibility levels in the family's interaction patterns may explain some of the differences in the family's response to demands. Specifically, ''flexibly-connected'' families seemed to be more vulnerable to the accumulation of stressful events, while ''structurally-separated'' families were affected more by transitional changes. ''Flexibly-separated'' and ''structurally-connected'' families, however, were affected by both transitions and stressful events. Therefore, the impact of events and transitions on family relationships was not determined by either the family's level of cohesion alone or the family's level of flexibility alone, but rather by some interaction of the two dimensions. Thus, while structural relations between variables were similar in all four types, other effects could be accounted for by the type of system, demonstrating the differential stress-coping processes in various types of families.

The results clearly indicated that well-being is influenced by the family's

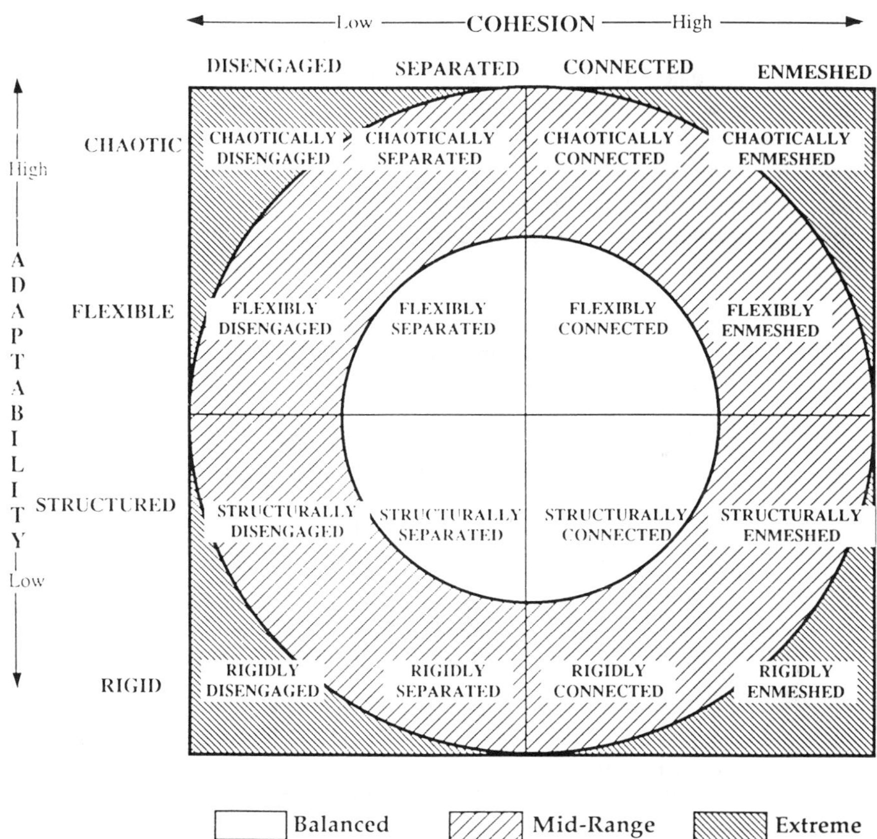

FIGURE 3 Circumplex model of family systems.

system type. That is, families with different interactional patterns, defined by cohesion in conjunction with adaptability, are influenced in different ways by the accumulations of life events and transitions and cope differently with these life stressors and strains.

LAZARUS AND FOLKMAN'S INTERDISCIPLINARY AND MULTILEVEL STRESS MODEL

Lazarus and Folkman's (1984) work at the Stress and Coping Project at Berkeley argues that research in stress, coping, and adaptation should be interdisciplinary and multileveled. They have developed a theory of stress and coping based on individual, cognitive psychology. While their research is primarily conducted from a psychological perspective, comprehensive investigations regarding stress should include interpretations that are social, psychological, and physiological. They therefore proposed the interdisciplinary, multilevel model for studying stress shown in Figure 4.

The process analysis of change over a period of time is illustrated by the move from immediate effects to long-term effects in the model. This model places adaptation on a continuum that includes three levels of functioning: the physical, psychological, and social levels of related health outcomes. These three levels are in turn related to three major long-term adaptational outcomes:

	Casual Anteedents	*Mediating Processes*	*Immediate Effects*	*Long-term Effects*
Social	SES Cultural Templates Institutional Systems Group Structures (eg. role patterns) Social Networks	Social supports as proferred Available social/ insititutional means of amiliorating problems	Social Disturbances Government responses Sociopolitical pressures Group Alienation	Social failure Revolution Social Change Structural Changes
Psychological	**Person variables:** values-commitments beliefs-assumptions, eg, personal control cognitive-coping style **Environmental:** (Situational) **variables:** situational demands imminence timing ambiguity social and material resources	Vulnerabilities Appraisal-Reppraisal **Coping:** problem-focused emotion-focused cultivating, seeking & using social support **Perceived social support:** emotional, tangible informational	Positive or negative feelings Quality of outcome of stressful encounters	Morale Functioning in the world
Physiological	Genetic or consiti-tutional factors Physiological conditioning Individual response Stereotypy Illness risk factors eg. smoking	Immune resources Species vulnerability Temporary vulnerability Acquired defects	Somatic changes (precursors of illness) Acute illness	Chronic illness Impaired physiological functioning Recovery from illness Longevity

FIGURE 4 Interdisciplinary and multilevel model of stress. From *Stress, Appraisal, and Coping* by Lazarus and Folkman, 1984. New York: Springer Publishing Company, Inc. Copyright 1984. Used by permission.

Somatic health and the physiological changes generated by stressful encounters; morale and the negative or positive effect a person may have both during and after stressful encounters; and social functioning, or a range of effectiveness with which demands from stressful encounters are managed. This more comprehensive model allows for interdisciplinary and multilevel research that can include, if desired, social and physiological levels as well as the psychological level. While this is a proposal for an interdisciplinary study of stress, it can serve a beginning point for the construction of a similar model that can examine health behaviors of individuals and families at a number of levels.

MULTISYSTEM ASSESSMENT OF STRESS AND HEALTH (MASH MODEL)

The results of this study and the studies reviewed by Campbell (1986) and Turk and Kerns (1985) suggest that a multidisciplinary model is needed if one is to adequately account for not only individual but also family system variables in the study of family behavioral health. An integrated system model developed by David Olson and Kenneth Stewart would take into account individual sources of stress, coping, and adaptation, and marital, family, and work "system" levels as well (see Figure 5).

The Multisystem Assessment of Stress and Health (MASH) model builds on the earlier models and research by Hill (1949); Hanson and Hill (1964); McCubbin and Patterson (1982, 1983); Pearlin and Schooler (1978); Pearlin, Menaghan, Lieberman, and Mullan (1981); Kanner, Coyne, Schaefer, and Lazarus (1981); Lazarus and Folkman (1984); and DeLongis (1985). Such a multisystem model provides for a more comprehensive examination of stressors and strains, and the subsequent level of adaptation. These stressors and strains, coping behaviors, and adaptational outcomes are examined in the four most common places of everyday living: one's personal life, marriage, family life, and work. The results of such a comprehensive assessment as this will allow the individual to better identify the sources of stressors and strains in his or her life, what resources he or she brings to bear in coping with those strains, and how healthy he or she is as a result.

The MASH Model enables one to deal with the significant questions proposed by Lazarus and Folkman (1984, p. 191). They suggested studying the impact of one role (i.e., work) on another role (i.e., marriage) and the direction of the influence. For example, does high job satisfaction positively affect the marriage (Kanter, 1977; Macoby, 1976; Seidenberg, 1973) and/or does the family help one cope with stress at work (Burke & Weir, 1979; House, 1979)?

The MASH Model proposed here hypothesizes that there are four system levels that need to be taken into account when examining stress and adaptation. Likewise, there are resources at each of these system levels that help buffer the

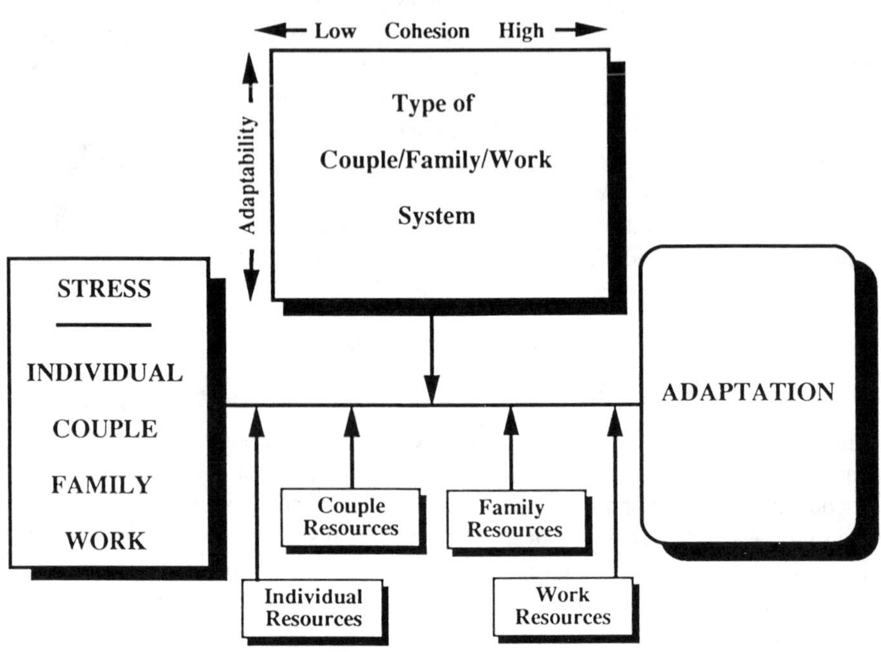

FIGURE 5 Multisystem Assessment of Stress and Health (MASH) model.

impact of stress on adaptation. This model would contain many of the elements proposed by Lazarus' interdisciplinary, multilevel model in Figure 4.

Four basic hypotheses that stem from the model are currently being tested in research conducted at the University of Minnesota.

- *Hypothesis No. 1. Stress has a negative impact on the level of overall adaptation.* This is the most fundamental hypothesis of the integrated model. It will examine whether and the degree to which each level of stress impacts the individual's overall adaptation.
- *Hypothesis No. 2. Individual, couple, family, and work resources will enable individuals to more adequately cope with stress and thus have higher levels of overall adaptation.* This hypothesis adds resources at each level in order to examine the degree to which individual, marital, family, or work resources mediate the impact of stress from each of the same four levels. Resources will be examined both within each level and between each level in order to determine which resources best mediate stress from which level. For instance, will marital resources be found to be an important mediator between work stress and overall individual adaptation? Or will the individual resource of self-esteem be found to be an important variable mediating between work

stress and individual adaptation or between marital strains and individual adaptation?

- *Hypothesis No. 3. Individuals in marital and family systems with high cohesion and adaptability will more adequately cope with stress and thus have higher levels of overall adaptation than individuals in marital and family systems with low cohesion and adaptability on the Circumplex Model.* This hypothesis will examine the extent to which the marital or family system (as conceptualized in the Circumplex Model) mediates between each of the four levels of stress and overall individual adaptation. Previous research has found a positive linear relationship between the two dimensions of cohesion and adaptability and well-being for nonclinical families. While it might be expected that individuals in more flexible and more cohesive systems will have fewer marital or parental strains, this study will also examine whether individuals will cope better with daily hassles or work stress than persons in less flexible and less cohesive systems.
- *Hypothesis No. 4. Individuals who are high in resources and have a marital or family system high in cohesion and adaptability will have higher levels of overall adaptation than individuals low in resources and in marital or family systems low in cohesion and adaptability, given the same amount of stress.* The fourth hypothesis represents the final integrated model of stress and adaptation that will be tested in this study. It will examine the extent to which resources both within and between each system level and the marital or family system type mediate the impact of stress upon overall individual adaptation.

In order to assess the various dimensions at the four system levels proposed by the MASH Model, an assessment tool called the *Health and Stress Profile* was recently developed by David Olson, Kenneth Stewart, and Lance Wilson. The specific scales for the HSP are listed in Figure 6.

The MASH Model enables one to examine which resources at the individual, marital, family, or work levels might buffer stressors and strains from the same or other levels. For example, would the resources of high self-esteem and a high degree of emotional expression buffer the stress from one's work more or less so than, say, a highly functional marital or family system? In other words, do marital and family system resources help buffer the impact of stressors and strains from work? Or, to what extent might strains from work affect the level of marital satisfaction?

These and many other questions might better be addressed if one begins with a more comprehensive assessment of the individual in the context of the systems in their life. Each of these systems has impacts on the level of stress and strains, as well as on the level of well-being. Sometimes the particular dysfunctioning of a system might create or further exacerbate strains for the individual, result in deteriorating physical or mental health. On the other hand,

		Individual	Work	Couple	Family
STRESS		Personal Stress 50 Psychological Distress 10 Physical Symptoms 20 Global Stress	Work Stress 28	Couple Stress 20	Family Stress 20
COPING RESOURCES	WHAT YOU DO	Problem Solving 7 Exercise Habits 5 Eating Habits 10 Alcohol/ Smoking (-) 12	Work Coping Style 6	Couple Coping Style 10	Family Coping Style 10
	WHAT YOU BELIEVE	Self-esteem 10 Mastery 7 Spiritual Beliefs 10		Social Desirability 5	
	YOUR RELATION-SHIP WITH OTHERS	Preferred Closeness 10 Preferred Flexibility 10 Emotional Expression 10 Social Support 10	Work Closeness 10 Work Flexibility 10 Work Communication 10	Couple Closeness 10 CoupleFlexibility 10 Couple Communication 10	Family Closeness 10 Family Flexibility 10 Family Communication 10
SATISFACTION		Personal Satisfaction 10	Work Satisfaction 10	Couple Satisfaction 10	Family Satisfaction 10
		195 Items	**74 Items**	**75 Items**	**70 Items**

TOTAL: 414 Items

FIGURE 6 Health and Stress Profile (HSP): An Overview.

when the family or work system is functioning well, these systems can serve as a highly significant resource for the individual.

CONCLUSION

This overview has examined a number of studies linking family systems to the individuals' mental and physical health. Studies in behavioral medicine, health psychology, and medical sociology have begun moving away from the traditional medical model and moving more in the direction of adapting a family systems paradigm as the principal framework by which health promotion programs, health behavior, and illness and stress behavior are examined. These efforts have produced a number of family theories and subsequent family assessments that attempt to measure family system properties. These assessments have in turn been applied to studies of family stress, family illness, and family health behavior.

The MASH Model is proposed to offer a more comprehensive assessment of stress, coping resources and behaviors, and adaptation at the four system levels: the individual, family, marital, and work systems. The need to include more than one system in the diagnosis and treatment of physical illness was recently proposed by Dym (1987), who recommends applying cybernetic concepts to the study of physical illness. A unified biopsychosocial field is assumed to supersede previous designations of illnesses as being merely "physical" or "psychological." Illness must be located in the ongoing interactions among biochemical, psychological, and social experiences. Dym argues that designating an illness as "physical" is an arbitrary punctuation of the larger field. A biopsychosocial model would allow for diagnosis and treatment in a more holistic framework. Dym's proposal of a biopsychosocial model and the development of and future research using the MASH Model are attempts to move beyond previous linear medical models. It is hoped that a multisystem cybernetic model will provide a more heuristic approach to understanding the relationship between the family and health behavior.

REFERENCES

Angell, R. (1936). *The family encounters the depression.* New York: Charles Scribner & Sons.

Antonovsky, A. (1987). *Unraveling the mystery of health.* San Francisco: Jossey-Bass.

Ashton, N. J. (1983). *Relationship of chronic physical activity levels to physiological and anthropometric variables in 9–10 year old girls.* Paper presented at the annual meeting of the American College of Sports Medicine, Montreal.

Baer, P. E., Reed, J., Bartlett, P. C., Vincent, J. P., Williams, B. J., & Bourianoff, G. G. (1983). Studies of gaze during induced conflict in families with a hypertensive father. *Psychosomatic Medicine, 45,* 233–242.

Baer, P. E., Vincent, J. P., Williams, B. J., Bourianoff, G. G., & Bartlett, P. C. (1980). Behavioral response to induced conflict in families with a hypertensive father. *Hypertension* (2, Suppl.), 1-70–1-77.

Baranowski, T., Chapin, J., & Evans, M. (1982). *Dimensions of social support for hypertension regimen compliance.* Galveston: University of Texas Medical Branch.

Baranowski, T., & Nader, P. R. (1985). Family health behavior. In D. Turk & R. D. Kerns (Eds.), *Health, illness and families.* New York: John Wiley & Sons.

Barnes, H., & Olson, D. H. (1985). Parent–adolescent communication and the Circumplex Model. *Child Development, 56,* 438–447.

Beavers, W. R., & Voeller, M. N. (1983). Family models: Comparing and contrasting the Olson Circumplex Model with the Beavers Systems Model. *Family Process, 22,* 250–260.

Becker, M. H., Drachman, R. H., & Kirscht, J. P. (1972). Predicting mothers' compliance with pediatric medical regiments. *Journal of Pediatrics, 81,* 843–854.

Becker, M. H., Drachman, R. H., & Kirscht, J. P. (1974). A new approach to explaining sick-role behavior in low-income populations. *American Journal of Public Health, 64,* 205–216.

Becker, M. H., & Green, L. W. (1975). A family approach to compliance with medical treatment: A selective review of the literature. *International Journal of Health Education, 18,* 2–11.

Benjamin, L. (1974). Structural analysis of social behavior. *Psychological Review, 81,* 392–425.

Benjamin, L. (1977). Structural analysis of a family in therapy. *Journal of Counseling and Clinical Psychology, 45,* 391–406.

Brownell, K. D. Heckerman, C. L., Westlake, R. J., Hayes, S. C., & Monti, P. M. (1978). The effects of couples training and partner co-operativeness in the behavioral treatment of obesity. *Behavioral Research and Therapy, 16,* 323–333.

Brownell, K. D., Kelman, J. H., & Stunkard, A. J. (1983). Treatment of obese children with and without their mothers: Changes in weight and blood pressure. *Pediatrics, 71,* 515–523.

Buckley, W. (1967). *Sociology and modern systems theory.* Englewood Cliffs, NJ: Prentice Hall.

Burke, R. J., & Weir, T. (1979). Patterns in husbands' and wives' coping behavior. *Psychological Reports, 44,* 951–956.

Campbell, T. L. (1986). *Family's impact on health: A critical review and annotated bibliography* (NIMH Series DN No. 6, DHHS Pub. No. [ADM] 86–1461). Washington, DC: U.S. Government Printing Office.

Charney, E., Bynum, R. Eldredge, D., Frank, D., Macy-Whinney, J. B., McNabb, N., Schneider, A., Sumpter, E. A., & Iker, H. (1967). How well do patients take oral penicillin? A collaborative study in private practice. *Pediatrics, 40,* 188–195.

Constantine, L. (1977, October). *A verified system theory of human process.* Paper presented at University of Minnesota Conference on Family Social Science.

Cromwell, R. E. Olson, D. H., & Fournier, D. G. (1976). Diagnosis and evaluation in marital and family counseling. In D. H. Olson (Ed.), *Treating relationships.* Lake Mills, Iowa: Graphic Publishing.

Cromwell, R. E., & Peterson, G. W. (1983). Multisystem multimethod family assessment in clinical context. *Family Process, 22,* 147–163.

DeLongis, A. (1985). *The relationship of everyday stress to health and well-*

being: Inter- and intraindividual approaches. Unpubl
tation. University of California, Berkeley.

Dent, O., & Goulston, K. (1982). Community attitudes t
Biosocial Science, 14, 359–372.

Diamond, E. L. (1982). The role of anger and hostility ir
sion and coronary heart disease. *Psychological Bulleti*

Doherty, W. J., Schrott, H. G., Metcalf, L., & Iasiello-vailas, L. (1983). Effect of spouse support and health beliefs on medication adherence. *Journal of Family Practice, 17,* 837–841.

Dym, B. (1987). The cybernetics of physical illness. *Family Process, 1,* 35–48.

Elling, R., Whittemore, R., & Green, M. (1960). Patient participation in a pediatric program. *Journal of Health and Human Behavior, 1,* 183–191.

Epstein, N. B., Baldwin, L., & Bishop, D. (1983). The McMaster Family Assessment Device. *Journal of Marital and Family Therapy, 9,* (2), 171–180.

Francis, V., Korsch, B. M., & Morris, M. J. (1969). Gaps in doctor–patient communication: Patients' response to medical advice. *New England Journal of Medicine, 280,* 535–540.

French, A. P., & Guidera, B. J. (1974). *The family as a system in four dimensions: A theoretical model.* Paper presented at Academy of Child Psychiatry, San Francisco.

Gath, A., Smith, M., & Baum, J. (1980). Emotional, behavioral and educational disorders in diabetic children. *Archives of Disease in Childhood, 55,* 371–375.

Goldstein, R. K., Gerhardt, P. R., & Handy, V. H. (1957). Some factors related to delay in seeking diagnosis for cancer symptoms. *Cancer, 10,* 1–7.

Gottman, J. M. (1979). *Marital interaction.* New York: Basic Books.

Hanson, D. A., & Hill, R. (1964). Families under stress. In H. Christensen (Ed.), *Handbook of marriage and the family.* Chicago: Rand McNally.

Hanson, D. A., & Johnson, V. A. (1979). Rethinking family stress theory: Definitional aspects. In W. R. Burr, R. Hill, F. I. Nye, & I. Reiss (Eds.), *Contemporary theories about the family* (Vol. I). New York: The Free Press.

Hartz, A., Giefer, E., & Rimm, A. A. (1977). Relative importance of the effect of family environment and heredity on obesity. *Annals of Human Genetics, 41,* 185–193.

Heinzelmann, F., & Bagley, R. W. (1970). Response to physical activity programs and their effects on health behavior. *Public Health Report, 85,* 905–911.

Hill, R. (1949). *Families under stress.* Westport, CT: Greenwood Press.

Hill, R. (1958). Generic features of families under stress. *Social Casework, 39,* 139–150.

..., J. S. (1979). Occupational stress and coronary heart disease: A review and theoretical integration. *Journal of Health and Social Behavior, 15,* 12–27.

Julius, M., Harburg, E., Cottington, E. M., & Johnson, E. H. (1987). Anger-coping types, blood pressure, and all-cause mortality: A follow-up in Tecumseh, Michigan (1971–1983). *American Journal of Epidemiology, 115,* 27–34.

Kanner, A. D., Coyne, J. C., Schaefer, C., & Lazarus, R. S. (1981). Comparisons of two models of stress measurement: Daily hassles and uplifts versus major life events. *Journal of Behavioral Medicine, 4,* 1–39.

Kanter, R. M. (1977). *Work and family in the United States: A critical review and agenda for research and policy.* New York: Russell Sage Foundation.

Kantor, D., & Lehr, W. (1975). *Inside the family.* San Francisco: Jossey-Bass.

Khoury, P., Morrison, J. A., Laskarzewski, P. M., & Glueck, D. J. (1983). Parent–offspring and sibling body mass index association during and after sharing of common household environments: The Princeton School District Family Study. *Metabolism, 32,* 82–89.

King, R. A., & Leach, J. E. (1951). Habits of medical care. *Cancer, 4,* 221–225.

Kleges, R. C., Coates, T. J., Moldenhauer, L. M., Holzer, B., Gustavson, J., & Barnes, J. (in press). The FATS: An observational system for assessing physical activity in children and associated parent behavior. *Behavioral Assessment.*

L'Abate, L. (1985). *The emporer has no clothes! Long live the emporer! A critique of family systems thinking and a reductionist proposal.* Unpublished manuscript.

Lavee, Y., McCubbin, H. I., & Olson, D. H. (1987). The effect of stressful life events and transitions on family functioning and well being. *Journal of Marriage and the Family, 49,* 857–873.

Lavee, Y., Olson, D. H., & McCubbin, H. I. (1988). *Family system types and adaptational outcomes: A challenge to stress theory.* Unpublished paper. Family Social Science, University of Minnesota.

Lazarus, R. S., & Folkman, S. (1984). *Stress, appraisal, and coping.* New York: Springer Publishing Company.

Leary, T. (1957). *Interpersonal diagnosis or personality.* New York: Ronald Press.

Leff, J., & Vaughn, C. (1985). *Expressed emotion in families.* New York: Guilford Press.

Leventhal, J., Leventhal, E. A., & Nguyen, T. V. (1985). Reactions of families to illness: Theoretical models and perspectives. In D. Turk, & R. D. Kerns (Eds.), *Health, illness and families.* New York: John Wiley & Sons.

Lewis, J. M., Beavers, R., Gossett, J. T., & Phillips, V. A. (1976). *No single thread: Psychological health in family systems.* New York: Brunner/Mazel.

Litman, T. J. (1974). The family as a basic unit in health and medical care: A social-behavioral overview. *Social Science and Medicine, 8,* 495–519.

Macoby, M. (1976). *The gamesman.* New York: Simon & Schuster.

McCubbin, H. I., & Patterson, J. M. (1982). Family adaptations to crisis. In H. I. McCubbin, A. Cauble, & J. Patterson (Eds.), *Family stress, coping and social support* (pp. 26–47). Springfield, IL: Charles C Thomas.

McCubbin, H. I., & Patterson, J. M. (1983). The family stress process: The Double ABCX model of adjustment and adaptation. In H. I. McCubbin, M. B. Sussman, & J. M. Patterson (Eds.), *Social stress and the family: Advances and developments in family stress theory and research* (pp. 7–73). New York: Haworth Press.

Mechanic, D. (1979). The stability of health and illness behavior: Results from a 16 year follow up. *American Journal of Public Health, 69,* 1142–1145.

Moos, R. (1974). *Manual for the family, work and group environment scales.* Palo Alto, CA: Consulting Psychologists Press.

Moos, R. H., & Moos, B. S. (1981). *Family environment scale manual.* Palo Alto, CA: Consulting Psychologists Press.

Nader, P. R., Baranowski, T., Vanderpool, N., Dworkin, R. J., & Dunn, K. (1983). The Family Health Project: Cardiovascular risk reduction education for children and parents. *Developmental and Behavioral Pediatrics, 4,* 3–10.

Olson, D. H. (1986). Circumplex Model VII: Validation Studies and FACES III. *Family Process, 25,* 337–351.

Olson, D. H. (1987). Assessment of family functioning. *NIDA research scales.* Washington, DC: National Institute on Drug Abuse.

Olson, D. H., Fournier, D. G., & Druckman, J. M. (1986). Counselor's manual for PREPARE/ENRICH (rev. ed.). Minneapolis: PREPARE/ENRICH, Inc.

Olson, D. H., Portner, J., & Lavee, Y. (1985). Family adaptability and cohesion evaluation scales (FACES III). Published Monograph. Family Social Science, St. Paul, Minnesota: University of Minnesota.

Olson, D. H., Russell, C., & Sprenkle, D. (1983). Circumplex model VI: Theoretical update. *Family Process, 18,* 3–28.

Olson, D. H., Sprenkle, D., & Russell, C. (1979). Circumplex model of marital and family systems: Cohesion and adaptability dimensions, family types and clinical application. *Family Process, 8,* 3–27.

Parsons, T., & Bales, R. F. (1955). *Family socialization and interaction process.* Glencoe, IL: Free Press.

Pearce, J. W., LeBow, M. D., & Orchard, J. (1981). Role of spouse involvement in the behavioral treatment of overweight women. *Journal of Counseling and Clinical Psychology, 49,* 236–244.

Pearlin, L. I., Menaghan, E. B., Lieberman, M. A., & Mullan, J. T. (1981). The stress process. *Journal of Health and Social Behavior, 22,* 337–356.

Pearlin, L. I., & Schooler, C. (1978). The structure of coping. *Journal of Health and Social Behavior, 19,* 2–21.

Perrier Corporation. (1979). *Fitness in America. The Perrier study.* Great Water, NY: Author.

Pratt, L. (1976). *Family structure and effective health behavior: The energized family.* Boston: Houghton-Mifflin.

Reiss, D. (1981). *The family's construction of reality.* Cambridge: Harvard University Press.

Sackett, D. L., & Haynes, R. B. (1976). *Compliance with therapeutic regimens.* Baltimore: Johns Hopkins University Press.

Seidenberg, R. (1973). *Corporate wives: Corporate casualties?* New York: AMA-COM.

Simonds, J. (1977). Psychiatric status of diabetic youth matched with a control group. *Journal of the American Diabetes Association, 26,* 921–925.

Skinner, H. A, Steinauer, P. D, & Santa Barbara, J. (1983). The Family Assessment Measure. *Canadian Journal of Community Mental Health, 2,* 91–105.

Steidl, J. H., Finkelstein, F. O., Wexler, J. P., Feigenbaum, H., Kitsen, J., Kliger, A. S., & Quinlan, D. M. (1980). Medical condition, adherence to treatment regimens and family functioning. *Archives of General Psychiatry, 37,* 1025–1027.

Turk, D. C., & Kerns, R. D. (1985). *Health, illness and families.* New York: John Wiley & Sons.

von Bertalanffy, L. (1968). *General systems theory.* New York: Braziller.

Waxman, M., & Stunkard, A. J. (1980). Calorie intake and expenditure of obese boys. *Journal of Pediatrics, 96,* 187–193.

Wilson, G. T., & Brownell, K. (1978). Behavior therapy for obesity: Including family members in the treatment process. *Behavioral Therapy, 9,* 943–945.

World Health Organization. (1976). *Statistical indices of family health* (Report No. 589).

3

GOAL SYSTEMS AND HEALTH OUTCOMES ACROSS THE LIFE SPAN: A PROPOSAL

Paul Karoly

Arizona State University

INTRODUCTION

Health behaviors and their determinants are central concerns in contemporary health psychology (Feuerstein, Labbe, & Kuczmierczyk, 1986; Taylor, 1986). Among the complex actions related to health status are those that ostensibly protect or promote health (or reduce illness risk), such as seeking help, engaging in regular exercise, managing stress, and eating nutritious foods in reasonable amounts. Further, individuals engage in behaviors that are said to threaten or compromise health (or increase illness risk), such as smoking cigarettes, taking drugs, and operating an automobile injudiciously (speeding, drinking and driving, failing to use seat belts). Health-compromising behaviors sometimes represent the absence of health-protective action, but this is not always the case. Included among the key determinants of health promotion/health endangerment are cultural, social, and economic factors, and psychological factors such as "personality" and "attitude," knowledge and education, and the vagaries of decision-making, cost-benefit analysis, and problem solving (cf., Matarazzo, Weiss, Herd, Miller, & Weiss, 1984; Weinstein, 1988).

While new and intriguing data are compiled daily relating health behaviors to various classes of identified determinants, the field is far from being systematically plowed and cultivated. Notably, we lack a unified theoretical frame-

The writing of this chapter was supported, in part, by Grant PMH-39246-03 establishing the Preventive Intervention Research Center (PIRC) at Arizona State University. The author wishes to express his appreciation to Mary Redondo for her efforts in manuscript preparation.

work within which to organize our growing data base. And for a truly integrative model to emerge, a number of problematic complexities would have to be addressed.

First, the relation of health protective to health compromising behaviors within the same person does not appear to be highly consistent or predictable, as correlations among classes of health behavior are not very high. Further, overall health status does not seem readily traceable to patterns of health protective/health risk behavior (Harris & Guten, 1979).

Second, health protective and health compromising behaviors assume quite different social and personal meanings in physically healthy individuals versus those with perceptible symptoms of illness. For example, cigarette smoking *after* a heart attack seems particularly irrational relative to the merely "ill-advised" smoking activity of teenagers; and the search for understanding of blatantly self-destructive acts has led to the postulation of explanatory processes such as unconscious self-deception, automaticity, denial, distortions in time perspective, and other aspects of "bounded rationality" (cf. Lockard & Paulus, 1988; Weinstein, 1987).

Finally, the multiple, psychosocial determinants of health-relevant behavior must themselves be presumed to function differently (a) in the healthy, the diagnosably sick, and the somatizing well; (b) in children, adults, and the elderly; (c) under varying conditions of personal receptivity to both informational and affective input; and (d) under conditions of noncognitive (nondecisional) mediation of action. Clearly, any unifying theory built around the *content* of health protective versus illness engendering behaviors must be capable of organizing disciplinary diversity of considerable magnitude.

After reviewing theoretical and empirical data bearing on why people sometimes do and sometimes do not act in their own best interests vis-à-vis their health, Cleary (1987) recently concluded that the field may be pursuing the wrong kinds of questions.

> *It is my opinion that there is no solution. . . . instead of developing more elaborate predictive "models," we should be trying to understand the* meaning *of the behaviors to individuals and the* processes *involved in encoding the acting on information.* (p. 141, emphasis added)

I do not contend here that current research on contextual, attitudinal, or decisional influences on health practices is necessarily "wrong," but rather that there are yet untapped routes to knowledge. On the other hand, I concur with Cleary's (1987) call for meaning-centered and process-relevant research. Beyond this, I suggest that we can utilize different *units of analysis* and that we seek *indirect* as well as direct links from the person or the setting to various biophysical outcomes or states.

My interest in doing things differently is motivated partly by the inadequacy of existing predictive models, such as the Health Belief Model (Becker & Maiman, 1975). Nonetheless, it is quite possible that this model's predictive failures (e.g., Calnan & Moss, 1984) and the shortcomings of other models derive mainly from the insensitivity of existing measures and experimental designs—a situation which will likely be remedied by psychometric and experimental advances. However, even with improvements in measurement and modeling, the domain of health psychology should remain open to new modes of inquiry. The purpose of this chapter, then, is to offer just such a new direction as a complement to existing approaches.

MOTIVATION AND GOAL-CENTERED UNITS OF ANALYSIS

The existence of a motivation means that there exists (a more or less exact) idea of a goal.

Dietrich Dorner (1985)

To suggest that health behaviors of various kinds are *motivated* denotes in many circles that forces, both intrapsychic and environmental, contribute to their instigation, vigor, and persistence. Economic conditions, support networks, prohealth attitudes, decisional freedom, and the like can all be construed as sources of motivation to behave righteously as regards one's physical well-being. Similarly, the absence of motives or motivating (enabling) conditions or the presence of nonbeneficial instigatory factors can be invoked as explanations—usually after the fact—of health compromising activities. Motivation is therefore perhaps the single most used and least useful "explanatory" construct in health psychology, for it frequently does little more than reify and concretize a complex, unfolding process, whose contribution to health status may as often be collateral as linear and categorical.

Since I contend that health behavior is indeed motivated, I should begin by clarifying my use of the term. First, let me state my belief that for an act or set of acts to be motivated does not imply that motive forces either in the person or in the situation impel and guide the behaviors in question. Rather, motivation is an emergent process, reflecting the interdependent operation of a network of adaptive functions. Such a perspective is inherently representational, in that it presumes that we humans possess and use the capacity to construct models (symbolic representations) of the world, the self, and (importantly) the variable relations between self and world (cf. Johnson-Laird, 1988). Self, world, and self–world knowledge structures are higher-order regulators of behavior, providing people with the potential for integrating their past, present, and imagined futures (cf. also Cantor, Markus, Niedenthal, & Nurius, 1986).

For a viable applied psychology, however, a unit of analysis is needed that is less molar than broad-based cognitive representations or personality characteristics but more integrative than single behaviors, attitudes, traits, or drives. Defining a "middle-level" analytic unit in absolute terms is difficult, given the obvious contextual influence contributed by one's anchoring points. When compared with generalized dispositions toward action or the sum total of an individual's beliefs and experiences, units built around concepts of self, styles of self-presentation, or problem-solving abilities certainly seem middle level. However, these constructs are culturally conditioned and value-laden and tend not to possess the characteristics of what Little (1987a) has called *systemically integrative* units. To be systemic, units should be commensurable within the single case; should cut across the behavioral, affective, and cognitive domains; and should be "modular rather than fixed" (i.e., personally meaningful rather than tied to group norms). A unit based upon an individual's relationship to his/her incentives would appear to provide a practical, readily interpretable codification of self–world commerce (cf. also Klinger, 1975). Such a unit may be said to consist of a goal, its context, and the operations necessary for goal-attainment. Nuttin (1984) referred to these elemental constituents as the *behavioral process.* Ford (1987), who calls this unit a *behavioral episode,* provided perhaps the most complete definition. According to Ford (1987), a behavior episode (BE) involves

> *(a) some set of consequences toward which it is directed . . . (b) a variable pattern of activities . . . selectively organized with feedforward and feedback to try to produce these consequences; (c) a set of environmental circumstances within which and toward which the behavior is directed; and (d) a termination of the pattern. (p. 149)*

The termination (or disengagement) occurs either when the goal is achieved, internal or external events change the priorities and direct the person toward an alternative, or the person judges the goal to be (currently) unattainable. Finally, Ford (1987) postulates that BEs are represented cognitively as prototypes, which he terms *behavioral episode schemata* (BES).

The BE and/or BES is systematic, integrative, personally meaningful yet nomothetically approachable, developmentally relevant, and measurable. The goal-centered unit is, therefore, offered as a possible addition to the psychologically segregated analytic structures heretofore used in the field of health psychology to serve as moderators (or mediators) between the impact of life events (stressors, transitions, challenges, and the like) and various physical or mental health outcomes. From specific behaviors and cognitive appraisals to more molar attitudes, personality traits, biological predispositions, coping mechanisms, attributional styles, and/or social contingencies, singular moderators of the life events–illness relationship have been identified (cf. Gentry & Kobasa, 1984; Krantz & Glass, 1984). In the pages that follow I shall try to illustrate how an analysis of self-regulated goal pursuits over the life span can lead to new insights into the determinants of health protective and health compromising behaviors.

THE NATURE AND FUNCTION OF PERSONAL GOAL SYSTEMS

Folklore, literature, the mass media, and our everyday experience tells us that we are a goal-directed species and that the contents of our aspirations display both stability and change over time. Children's goals are immediate and immature. Young adults aspire to achieve and find a place for themselves. The elderly seek to redefine themselves and their roles in the light of changing circumstances (retirement, death of a spouse, etc.) and the decline of physical vigor. Indeed, an individual's understanding of self, world, and self–world relations is, to a large degree, written in the language of goals and preferences that are themselves the products of historically-situated interactions among people and of biogenetic constraints. Perhaps because of the joint physiologic and social constructionist origins of goals, the tendency among many social scientists has been to study them more as end points or categories than as processes and dynamic, directive mechanisms.

Consider, for example, Kuhlen's (1968; Kuhlen & Johnson, 1952) classic studies of goal changes during the adult years. Citing the work of Maslow and Lewin, Kuhlen traced the rise and fall of specific aspirations as a function of either goal satisfaction or goal frustration (anxiety and threat) under the general guidance of basic needs. The young adult years were seen to be dominated by "growth–expansion" motives, while the later years were said to come under the influence of anxiety "generated by physical and social losses" (Kuhlen, 1968, p. 131). In analytic schemes such as this (cf. also Veroff & Veroff, 1980), underlying *motives* or *values* take on the major explanatory power, with goal-directedness a derivative or outcome. While not wishing to slight such approaches, I contend simply that they are incomplete.

Using an automobile excursion as a metaphor for the life course, I view such models as destination- and fuel-centered, although they certainly recognize that road conditions will often play a key role. An expanded view focuses upon the vehicle and the journey itself and appears amenable to empirical analysis. The expanded framework inquires about the functional components of the human conveyance and its structural integrity, as well as about setting conditions that may slow it down or facilitate its trip. Instead of just asking what a person wants and why, the model shows that it is equally important to ask *how* a person wants.

The basic outline of the expanded viewpoint, with special emphasis upon its health implications, is depicted in Figure 1. Goal types, which have been the subject of early (e.g., Maslow, Lewin, and Erikson) and contemporary (e.g., Ford & Nichols, 1987; Little, 1983; Pervin, 1983; Wadsworth & Ford, 1983;

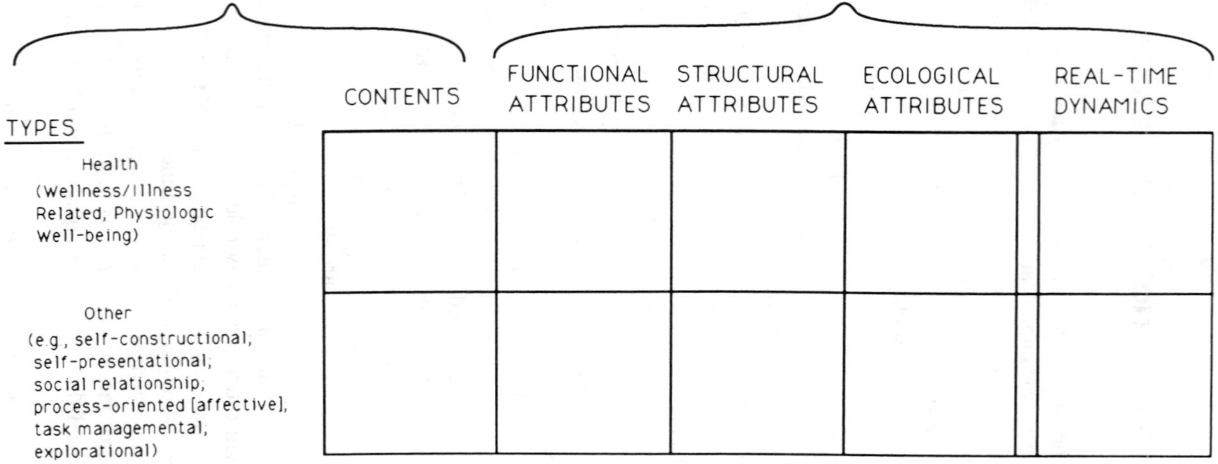

TYPES	CONTENTS	FUNCTIONAL ATTRIBUTES	STRUCTURAL ATTRIBUTES	ECOLOGICAL ATTRIBUTES	REAL-TIME DYNAMICS
Health (Wellness/Illness Related, Physiologic Well-being)					
Other (e.g., self-constructional; self-presentational; social relationship; process-oriented [affective]; task managemental; explorational)					

FIGURE 1 Goal types and goal attributes as descriptive and explanatory elements in a goal systems analysis.

Winell, 1987) analyses, are divided into *wellness/illness-related* and *other.* Attempts to organize goals into typologies have typically sought comprehensiveness either via a *surface features* approach (e.g., work, school, recreational, spiritual, and the like) or a more theoretical perspective. I have opted for a middle-level solution within which the pursuit of physiological well-being (health) is given special recognition along with categories that derive from action theory and contemporary cognitive social learning research (cf. Bandura, 1986; Baumeister, 1986; Csikszentmihalyi, 1975; Ford, 1987; Ford & Nichols, 1987; Klinger, 1975; Kuhl & Beckmann, 1985; Wicklund & Gollwitzer, 1982). Categories listed under "other" are viewed as very important heuristically, and are "secondary" only for present didactic purposes. Some will be discussed later in this chapter. For now, I maintain simply that the pursuit of health or avoidance of illness may be taken as a critical class of goals (destinations) differing, first, in terms of specific *content.*

Notwithstanding the descriptive value of goal types and contents, the remainder of the dimensions noted in Figure 1 provide the explanatory power; for, as noted by Pervin (1983), "it is the *movement toward goals* that gives behavior its organized, patterned quality" (p. 10).

Because goals are extended in time and space, enacted in the company of other people, and evoke emotions and evaluative reactions from the actor, they can be rated along a number of cognitive, behavioral, social, and affective dimensions. That is, in addition to knowing what a person wishes to achieve (e.g., to stop smoking cigarettes), we can inquire into the person's expectancies about goal attainment, perceptions of goal importance, attributions about loci of control, beliefs about behavioral enactment skills, and/or ratings of the positive/negative arousal associated with goal pursuit. The impact of the goal on others can also be assessed. Basically, these dimensions are capable of being functionally related to important outcomes, such as eventual goal attainment, academic achievement, mental health, life-satisfaction, and (especially in the current context) physical health status (cf. Cantor, Brower, & Korn, 1985; Emmons, 1986; Emmons & King, 198; Palys & Little, 1983; Ruehlman & Wolchik, 1988). Thus, I refer to organized collections of dimensions as *functional attributes* (see Figure 1).

Contemporary goal systems researchers have typically justified their choice of functional dimensions on the basis of common sense (the *importance* of a goal will surely make a difference in its pursuit), research (perceived *self-efficacy* usually predicts activity patterns), or theoretical concerns (competence in *planning* should enhance ultimate goal achievement). Little (1983) originally proposed 17 dimensions, Emmons (1986) employed 14 to 18 in his "Striving Assessment Scales," and Karoly, McKeeman, and Clapper (1985, November) used 26 dimensions (adding self-management items to those used by Little and his colleagues). Various attempts to reduce the list of functional dimensions through factor analysis have yielded several higher-order constructs: mastery, strain, and involvement (Ruehlman & Wolchik, 1988); meaning, structure, stressfulness, project efficacy, and sense of community (Little, 1987a); and degree of striving, success, ease, desirability, and instrumentality (Emmons, 1986).

Despite the advantage of the diagnostic flexibility that inheres in an "open" listing of functional goal dimensions, a conceptual organization of functional attributes (a higher-order construct) would permit greater comparability across investigations (although most researchers emply a core of very similar, if not identical, dimensions) and, more importantly, would strengthen the theoretical scaffolding of goal analytic research. I shall briefly outline a framework, based on the brilliantly integrative review of control theory models by Ford (1987), which I believe furnishes the needed systemization.

Instead of working up from lists of the cognitive, affective, or motor "properties" of goals, we can begin with a model of how complex living systems coordinate their components (a top-down approach). After reviewing the workings of mechanical, animal, and human control systems, Ford (1987) offered a conception of governing and arousal functions that helps to symbolize and organize diverse goal properties. As indicted in Figure 2, four key functions are the directive, the regulatory, the control, and the arousal function. The first three (called *governing functions*) allow an individual to make use of, store, transform, and organize information, thus providing "the centralized coordination that is necessary to maintain the flexibility and adaptability of complex systems" (Ford, 1987, p. 91). Diverse but interrelated forms of cognition are associated with each of the three governing functions.

The directive form of cognition is *end-state oriented,* reflecting the person's representations of goals and subgoals (e.g., What states or outcomes do I wish to bring about? How do I characterize my objectives?). Attributions about the importance of goals or the actor's skill at bringing them forth are clearly end-state cognitions, as are other generalizations the person makes about the attainment potential of his aspirations. Every goal researcher to date has included some directive functions on his or her list of dimensions. This functional attribute is also sometimes called a *feedforward function.* As Ford (1987) notes:

> *For a control system to be adaptive in a variable environment, it must be able to combine "current news" with "old news" to predict "future news." That ability would enable it to act not only in terms of what* has *happened but in terms of what is* likely *to happen.* (p. 68)

Desires, preferences, and anticipated possibilities push the system forward, in contrast to the more familiar *feedback function,* which Ford (1987) calls *regulatory.*

The regulatory function represents the monitoring of what the system has done and the evaluation of the match between desired reference values (or

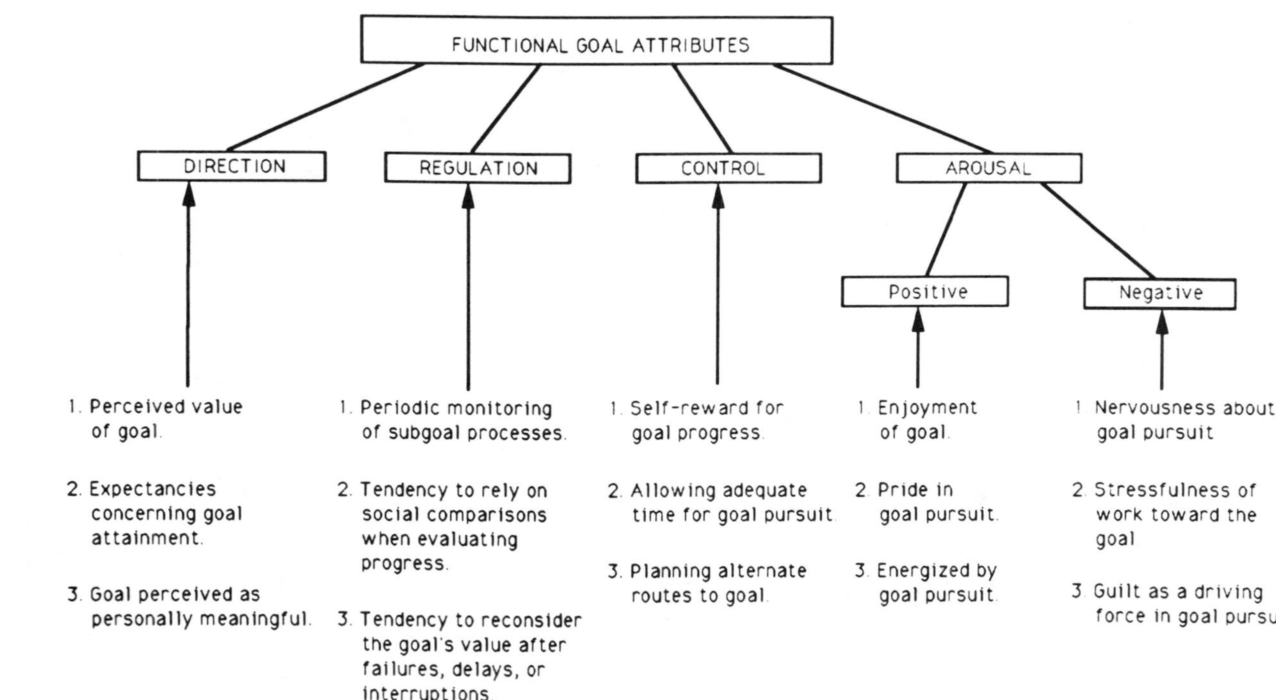

FIGURE 2 The Four Functional Attributes (from Ford, 1987) and some representative indicators (from the Goal Systems Interview).

standards) and input. Regulatory cognition is "cold" and process-evaluative (feedback-oriented, e.g., "What did I do and how well?").

To govern a complex system, action-guidance cognitions are also needed. Do I reward success and punish failure? Do I move toward my goals strategically and planfully? These are *control* cognitions and represent the third type of governing function (with motor skills as their behavioral counterpart).

Finally, for our purposes, a fourth function postulated by Ford (1987) needs to be included: the arousal function. Goal-directed living systems need to be activated, as all functioning requires energy to fuel both thought and action. Further, the activation process must be selective and variable in order to be responsive to changes in the external world. Ford (1987) has suggested that arousal (a term which is often used synonymously with motivation) is of two types: one type that energizes the nervous system to deal with (i.e., collect, transform, and use) information, and another that energizes overt action. Since the present system is geared only to deal with self-reported cognitions concerning mood, it reflects the selectivity and responsivity aspects of affect rather than its target. Following Watson, Clark, and Tellegen's work (Watson, 1988; Watson & Clark, 1984; Watson, Clark, & Tellegen, 1988; Watson and Tellegen, 1985), two independent factors are utilized to capture the dominant dimensions of self-rated emotional experience. The first, *positive affect,* is said to reflect an individual's "level of pleasurable engagement" with the world (often labeled pleasantness–unpleasantness or extraversion). The second, *negative affect,* is a "subjective distress" dimension (also called arousal and anxiety/neuroticism). To my knowledge, this is the first application of the two-factor model to the characterization of goal appraisals.

In sum, the four functional attributes I have included in the model of goal directiveness are designed to capture more of the necessary components of effective control systems than has heretofore been the case. Ford's (1987) approach, unlike many extant "control theory" conceptions, includes the variable energy source needed to drive the governing functions, extends beyond the directive function in characterizing goal cognitions (compare with Emmons' [1986] 18 dimensions, which are predominantly end-state cognitions), and includes both the feedback and the feedforward capacities. For reasons not entirely clear, prominent goal theorists have tended to emphasize one of the governing functions over the others (e.g., Bandura [1986] stresses the feedforward self-efficacy attribution, Carver & Scheier [1981] the regulatory feedback process, and Kuhl [1985] the control-related "action-state orientation").

It is not only comprehensiveness that attaches to the functional control systems perspective, but its ability to transcend the evanescence of particular goal objects in our day-to-day lives. What particular goals are being sought by an individual or what basic needs are being served may be less revealing than the framework within which goals are organized. Further, the presumed consistency of goal attributes may reflect the stable aspects of "personality," which have been so hotly contested in recent years (cf. Pervin, 1983). Finally, one can point to the potential utility of the four-fold functional attribute conception for the purpose of clinical assessment (i.e., pinpointing a deficit in the directive, regulatory, or control function) and for clinical intervention (i.e., the need, respectively, for values classification, cognitive restructuring, or problem-solving training).

Perhaps even more likely to remain consistent over long periods is the next category of explanatory construct, the *structural attributes*. I conceive of structural attributes as second-order, in that they represent ways of characterizing the content dimension. Three types of structural attributes, derived mainly from the social cognition and cognitive learning literatures, are assessed. These include (a) goal complexity, (b) goal conflict, and (c) domain specificity/generality. While space limitations prevent a comprehensive review of each of these structural attributes, their fundamental relevance to goal systems and their empirical contributions will be briefly reviewed.

Goals as standards or reference signals in a control system do not exist in isolation, but rather are believed to form an articulated network of self-directive cognitions. The network is typically described as a *hierarchy.* Unfortunately, the hierarchy notion is highly content bound, with some goals actually representing superordinate values (e.g., to be a respected person) and others representing subordinate values (e.g., to win a trophy in a particular sport). While superset–subset relations are important, assessing this dimension is time-consuming and taxing on research participants. A second aspect of organization, however, is not only practical but also important to the *efficiency* of the structural network. Complexity of goals, as indexed by their distinctiveness (attribute differentiation) is a measure of system interdependence or relatedness (cf. Emmons, 1989; Ford, 1987). Goal complexity is assessed by having subjects or clients sort their goals into as many distinct groups as desired and then calculating redundancy (vs. distinctiveness) by means of the information theory statistic, H (cf. Linville, 1987; Scott, Osgood, & Peterson, 1979). The greater the goal complexity, the greater the "equifinality" of the system, allowing the individual to select alternate paths to valued incentives (cf. Winell, 1987).

Perhaps the most widely studied structural dimension is *goal conflict.* Conflict per se is viewed as a basic requirement of all living systems, since control theory is built upon the presumption that a mismatch between valued reference standards and current conditions (input) is highly likely in variable environments. Only a system that lives and develops in a changeless, obstacle-free world can avoid having to deal with disturbances to its equilibrium. On the other hand, conflict *among* goals in a system with multiple reference values is not inevitable; nor is it desirable. Furthermore, even in a system with nonconflicting goals, disruption can occur if plans or problem-solving routines are incompatible (Miller, Galanter, & Pribram, 1960). In his Personal Projects

Analysis method, Little (1983, 1987b) applies what he calls a *secondary analysis* to determine how individual projects or goals impact (for better or worse) upon each other. Using a procedure very similar to Little's *cross-impact matrix,* Emmons and King (1988) found that conflict among strivings was related not only to psychological outcomes (such as negative affect and depression) but also to physical health indices (such as somatization, number of illnesses, and number of health center visits). Conflict is assessed (by the present author and others) through the use of systematic pairings of each goal on a subject's list with every other goal and the requirement that a rating reflective of helpfulness to obstructiveness be made for each pair. Note that the ratings need not be symmetric (i.e., if goal 1 is seen as conflicting highly with the pursuit of goal 2, the reverse will not necessarily be the case).*

The last structural attribute to be considered here is domain specificity versus domain generality in the pursuit of personal projects or goals. Just as goal complexity is hypothesized to serve as a buffer against specific failures or delays in strivings, so too is having a wide array of domains being pursued (domain generality). Following Linville's (1985) work, which suggests that "putting all your eggs in one cognitive basket" can produce affective disruption, we anticipate that having a variety of goal targets limits the degree of disheartenment which occurs when roadblocks are encountered in any single aspirational area. Employing a goal content categorizing system with sufficient scope to encompass most of an individual's stated goals (such as Little's [1983] system or that of Ford and Nichols [1987]), the specificity/generality metric denotes the number of distinct categories into which a participant's goals are assigned by a trained rater (e.g., when eliciting at least 10 active goals, the metric can vary between 1 and 10).

It would be a serious mistake to study goal pursuits without considering the role of environmental (setting) factors. The third type of explanatory construct in the goal systems approach (see Figure 1), *ecological attributes,* refers to the individual's perceptions regarding the degree to which each of his or her goals is supported by significant others and hindered (or impeded) by significant others. For each goal listed, then, participants indicate both the amount and quality of the available support, as well as the amount of interference encountered (a total of three separate ratings). While the effects of social support as a potential moderator of life stress and adaptation are by now well known (cf. Cohen & Wills, 1985; Lin, Dean, & Ensel, 1986; Sarason & Sarason, 1985), the goal systems model provides for comprehensiveness (a) by allowing support to be measured in the context of other relevant aspects of psychosocial function-

*Emmons (e.g., Emmons & King, 1988) also assesses what he calls within-striving conflict (or ambivalence) by asking subjects to indicate how unhappy they might be if they succeeded at each goal on their list. In the present system, a directive function indicator ("How certain are you that this goal is in your best interests?") serves an equivalent function.

ing (the functional and structural dimensions) as recommended by Wallston, Alagna, DeVellis, and DeVellis (1983) and (b) by allowing for the independent assessment of hindrance, a dimension which is believed to be relatively independent of support and likewise to have significant impact on various aspects of adjustment (cf. Fiore, Becker, & Coppel, 1983; Rook, 1984; Ruehlman & Wolchik, 1988).

In the Goal Systems Interview (GSI), an assessment procedure currently being used and refined by the author in collaboration with Dr. Linda Ruehlman and various students, 11 functional, structural, and ecological attribute scores are derived from participants' responses to a series of questions, probes, sorting tasks, and listing and comparing exercises that require approximately 90 minutes to complete. Typically, subjects are asked prior to the interview to think about 10 to 20 important goals in their lives that are both current (active) and distinct. Such a procedure usually yields at least 10 goals that fit the above criteria and that can meaningfully be rated. Depending upon our analytic purpose, we may ask subjects to be particularly mindful of certain goal categories, for example, physical health and safety. However, generally, goal categorization is accomplished by trained raters after the GSI has been completed.

The flexibility of the goal systems analysis approach permits the study of direct linkages from health-relevant goals to health-related outcomes (such as medication compliance or cigarette smoking) or of indirect linkages from general goal attributes to health-relevant outcomes. Using large, known groups facilitates data analysis in several ways. For example, if we were working with a large population of dieters and knew which ones were currently losing weight and which were not, we could find, in each subject's list of goals, the most important health goal (which will usually be "to lose weight") and compare the known groups in terms of attribute or specific indicator differences (e.g., as noted in Figure 2, the Functional Attributes divide into 5 levels and these, in turn, have 6 indicators each, in the current version of the GSI). Self-efficacy is a directive function indicator that might be found to discriminate among the groups. Or perhaps a composite of high self-efficacy with low goal ambivalence (another directive function indicator) might be needed. Or the groups might differ not in their end-state cognitions, but rather in their regulatory habits. The value of the goal systems perspective is that many potentially important mediators or moderators can be examined relationally. In fact, with large groups, I recommend the use of configural or profile analyses (cf., Aldenderfer & Blashfield, 1984; Filsinger & Karoly, 1985). Figure 3 depicts three hypothetical patterns that might emerge from group data and that could prove useful in predicting physical health outcomes for particular target populations.

If a single population were available with a specific health outcome measurable on an interval scale (e.g., diabetics with values on glycosylated hemoglobin), the investigator could utilize multiple regression methods to determine goal systems components most strongly related to health status.

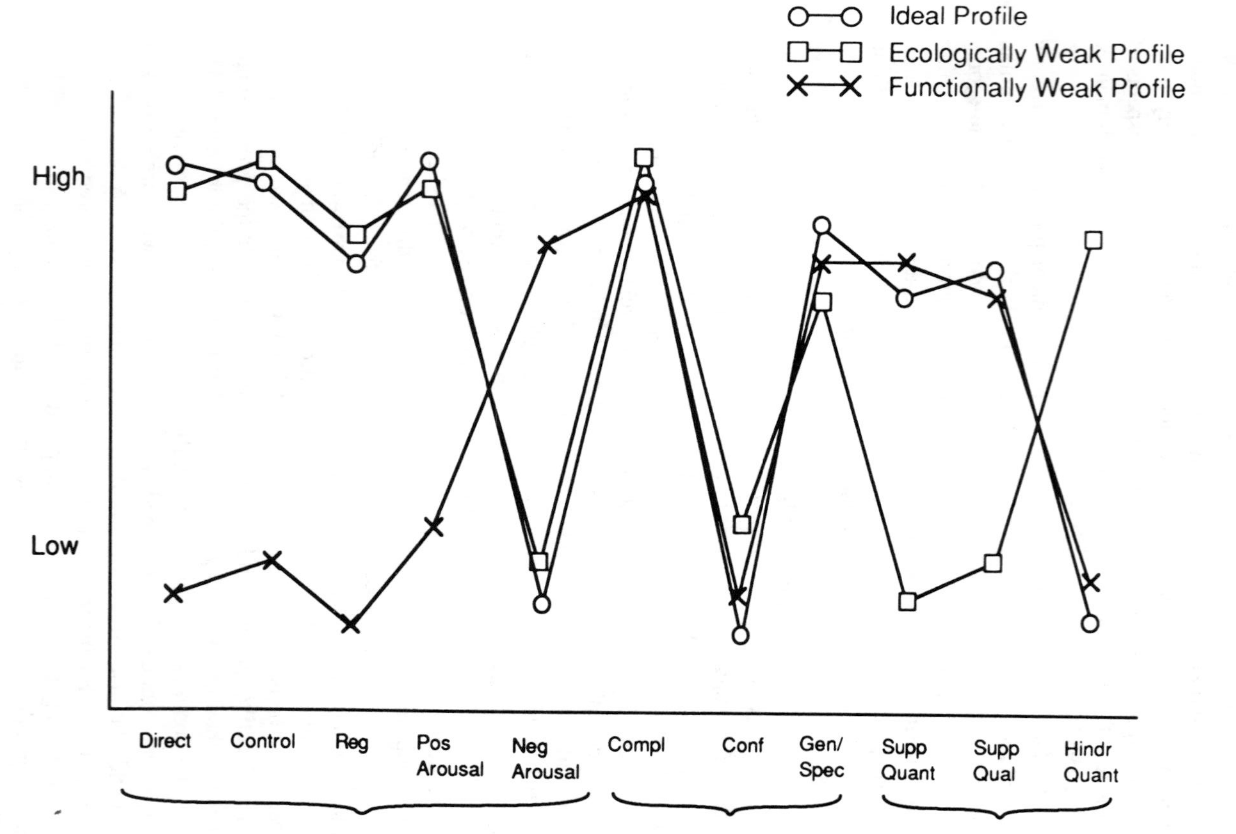

FIGURE 3 A set of hypothetical profile types from the Goal Systems Interview.

The present system also permits health goals to be compared with other hypothesized determinants of health outcome (e.g., beliefs, family variables, disorder-specific factors such as chronicity, doctor–patient relationship variables, etc.) in order to assess the comparative importance of motivational elements. Similarly, the role of *nonhealth goals* can be assessed in terms of the goals' organization across known groups or their absolute versus relative contribution to important health or illness endpoints.

GOAL SYSTEMS AND HEALTH: SOME GENERAL HYPOTHESES

It is my contention that the systematic organization of specific health goals will have important implications for those health activities and medical status variables that are directly goal-linked. That is, for the goal "to quit smoking," the attendant functional, structural, and ecological profile will play a significant, causal role in a person's eventual smoking status and, hence, in his or her risk of death due to lung cancer. This rather obvious and perhaps noncontroversial hypothesis has not yet been empirically tested at the systems level in any high risk domain such as cigarette smoking, alcoholism, drug addiction, or obesity. However, particular elements of the model (e.g., self-efficacy, which is one of the directive functions, and social support) have been shown to be predictive of long-range abstinence from certain health-threatening behaviors (cf. Bandura, 1986; Marlatt, 1985; Shumaker & Grunberg, 1986). Outcome studies using the GSI may well yield important new insights into the process of substance abuse treatment and relapse.

Health/illness outcomes, however, need not be contingent solely upon the integrity of systems of health-specific aspirations or strivings. The role of goal cognition in defining vocational performance objectives, in promoting self-perceptions of competence and mastery, in regulating interpersonal behavior, in helping to translate intentions into actions, in managing mood, and in helping to structure our discretionary time (away from work or school) points to the very real possibility that goal systems may link indirectly to physical health status (cf. Csikszentmihalyi & Larson, 1984; Elliott & Dweck, 1988; Klinger, 1975, 1982; Locke, Shaw, Saari, & Latham, 1981; Scheier & Carver, 1988). I therefore contend that general goal systems serve as a powerful yet neglected set of moderators of the relation between life stress and physical illness, between attitude–knowledge–belief structures and self-protective action (including compliance and health-care services utilization), and between chronic illness/disease states and subjective health outcomes (such as disability, pain, and demoralization). Some of the piecemeal evidence in support of my assertions will be presented next.

The Directive Function and Health

Because goals provide the reference standards around which self-directed behavior is organized, and since the instantiation of a particular goal in a free society assumes that it has been selected (often without awareness) from among alternative goals, we can view the directive function in expectancy–value terms. Extant goals-assessment procedures strongly emphasize the values aspect of end-state cognition by tapping into the "oughtness," necessity, and goodness–badness dimensions, such as importance, value, social desirability, relevance, and commitment. The expectancy aspect is represented by ratings of self-efficacy, outcome expectancy, probability of success, and the like (cf. Emmons, 1986; Feather, 1982; Little, 1983; Pervin, 1983). Since an individual can value and expect an outcome, state, or experience but see him- or herself as not having freely elected to engage its pursuit, the Goal Systems Interview also asks if the goal is imposed versus self-selected. Using a value × expectancy × origin definition of the directive function (or an expectancy × value model), it is easy to see why goal analyses based largely on directiveness tend to (a) help bridge the gap between various forms of knowledge and the likelihood of future action and (b) predict psychological functioning and life satisfaction.

The formal properties of (mainly directive) goal systems have repeatedly been shown to influence subjective well-being (Emmons, 1986; Palys & Little, 1983; Ruehlman & Wolchik, 1988). Typically, investigators employing similar lists of directive-function indicators have correlated either specific indicators or factor scores with such inventories as the Satisfaction With Life Scale (Diener, Emmons, Larsen, & Griffin, 1985) or the Mental Health Inventory (Veit & Ware, 1983) which yields a measure of psychological well-being and of distress. Palys and Little (1983) first found support for the general hypothesis that "the way people perceived, structured, and organized their project systems would be related to the satisfaction they felt with their lives as a whole" (p. 1227). Emmons (1986) had participants rate affect 4 times per day over a 3-week period and found that well-being as indexed by affect scores was highly correlated with goal importance, probability of success, and value. Thus, it can be asserted that the directive properties of goals should act as generalized stress buffers and, hence, demonstrate their relevance to health status.

One end-state (feedforward) cognition with an expectancy focus is self-efficacy. It is assessed in the GSI by asking participants to rate each of their goals in terms of the degree to which the respondent believes that he or she possesses the skills necessary to achieve the stated objective. Self-efficacy is a directive function indicator with strong empirical links to health. Bandura (1986) has reviewed research that shows, among other things, that cardiac patients' perceived physical efficacy predicts exercise compliance and "is a better predictor of resumption of an active life than cardiovascular capacity as reflected in peak heart rate on the treadmill" (p. 437). Further, data support the view that self-efficacy attributions can assist in pain tolerance, both in the laboratory and in real-life contexts such as childbirth (Manning & Wright, 1983) and arthritic pain (O'Leary, 1985). Finally, evidence exists to support the notion that self-efficacy underlies efforts to adopt health lifestyle practices (e.g., giving up cigarettes) and supports the maintenance of these practices over time (cf. also Marlatt, 1985).

Another indicator of end-state cognition on the GSI is the question that asks participants to indicate their degree of certainty that each goal on the list is "in your best interests." High scores on uncertainty for goals which are current and important indicate ambivalence. Interestingly, Emmons and King (1988) have shown that their measure of goal ambivalence is related to physical symptomatology (correlations in the .20 range; not significant with a 48-subject sample).

The GSI also asks participants to indicate the degree to which goals are chosen versus imposed (assuming that this isn't always a dichotomy). However, in a recent study in my laboratory (Karoly & Bay, 1988, August) we sought to investigate the implications of just such a dichotomy as perceived by young children. Specifically, 47 children between 10 and 18 years of age with Type I diabetes were asked to complete the Children's Personal Project Matrix (CHPPM), which included such directive function indicators as self-efficacy and importance, as well as 6 other functional goal attributes. However, children were first asked to sort a list of 21 diabetes-related self-care activities (goals) into three groups: "Things I do because I want to do them," "Things I do because someone else tells me to do them," and "Things I don't do." Six items each from the "told to do" and "want to do" sortings were then separately rated along 8 functional dimensions. Our purpose was to see if the factor structure of the ratings would differ across imposed versus self-selected goals, and if an important index of health (the amount of glucose in a blood assay) could be differentially predicted on the basis of functional attribute properties. We expected chosen ("want to do") goals would be a better predictor of glycosylated hemoglobin (metabolic control).

First, we found that children with diabetes could readily sort health-relevant goals into categories based upon degree of decisional freedom. More importantly, the factor structure of imposed goals differed from that of "want to do" goals (despite the fact that the same 8 indictors were being rated for both). The first factor for imposed goals was labeled *coercion,* whereas the first rotated self-selected goals factor was termed *mastery/enjoyment.* Most intriguing, however, was our finding that only imposed goal factors correlated with an assay measure of metabolic control. The higher the coercion (low self-efficacy, high upsettingness, high difficulty), the worse the metabolic control. However, dependency (low control, high importance) predicted good control. As far as the pursuit of diabetes "self-care" goals are concerned, it would appear that authoritative (not authoritarian) parents are probably the most potent source of goal-directedness in their children's lives.

The Regulatory Function and Health

The regulatory function consists of operating rules through which goal progress is monitored, standards are assessed, and evaluative judgments rendered. It is a feedback-sensitive and feedback-dependent set of appraisals. Although the regulatory function is fed by directive signals, it is the regulatory process that most reflects the "how" of self-directedness, capturing individual styles of thinking about self, about action, and about outcome. Importantly, it is the functional goal attribute most often omitted from extant goal assessment protocols.

Regulatory functions come immediately to mind when considering how general (non-health related) goals can influence health or moderate the stress–illness relation. Of the regulatory function indictors on the GSI, I shall focus on 2: the degree to which individuals tend to raise their standards after a successful movement toward the goal (success monitoring) and the degree to which individuals tend to lower their standards after delays or failures in goal pursuit (failure monitoring).

Failure monitoring of a self-defining goal, in combination with viewing the goal as important, having low perceived self-efficacy (two directive functions), and a tendency toward negative arousal (the arousal function) should predispose the actor to depression (compare with Pyszczynski & Greenberg's [1987] theory of self-regulatory perseveration). Depressive affect and performance retardation are very likely ingredients in the medical noncompliance equation or the failure to act upon one's knowledge of a "risky" situation.

Success monitoring can also be problematic when combined with deficiencies in the control function (e.g., poor time allotment and low rates of self-administered reward for success) (see Figure 2). Such a style may undergird the Type A (coronary-prone) pattern. Further, since many efforts to alter the Type A pattern focus on the directive function (i.e., trying to help patients modify their values and expectancies), the present systems view might explain the generally disappointing results of many Type A interventions (cf. Roskies, 1980).

Even when viewed in isolation from the other goal systems indicators (not a practice I endorse), the success and failure monitoring dimensions can be seen to resemble the constructs of *optimism* and *pessimism,* which are currently popular in the health psychology arena. Assuming a general equivalence between our GSI indicators and the questionnaire measure of dispositional optimism, the Life Orientation Test (LOT; Scheier & Carver, 1985), we might expect a similar relation of regulatory functions to coping styles and social-support seeking in stressful situations (cf. Scheier, Weintraub, & Carver, 1986).

Recall that the goals being monitored and evaluated in the regulatory cognitive mode are not necessarily health-relevant. Dysfunctional appraisal of social objectives (making friends, for example), self-esteem goals (e.g., to win a particular award), self-constructional goals (e.g., obtaining professional certification), process-oriented objectives (e.g., to get oneself relaxed before dinner), or task-oriented projects (like painting a room) can be disruptive to well-being, arouse negative feelings (anxiety, hostility, or depression), and, if prolonged, weaken the body's resistance to stress and disease.

Control and Arousal Functions and Health

Because Ford's (1987) classificatory system organizing the governing and arousal functions has not yet been used to distinguish so-called functional attributes, indirect evidence will again need to be mustered in support of my general hypotheses. However, both control (as an index of tactical or strategic cognition) and arousal (mood) have a history of association with medical outcome variables such as recovery from illness, regimen compliance, and service utilization. Control is our system's equivalent of coping, and arousal (positive and negative) taps the perhaps universal affective structure domain (level of pleasure vs. level of arousal). The literature on coping and health is quite large (see Lazarus & Folkman, 1984) and the role of positive and negative arousal (affect) in health has recently been discussed by Watson (1988).

However, to illustrate the goal systems application of control and arousal concepts, I will briefly note a study conducted in our laboratory (Karoly, McKeeman, & Clapper, 1985) which sought to extend Little's (1983) Personal Project Analysis methodology in the examination of self-change goals (weight loss and exercise) with obvious health implications. We noted, in a group of over 300 college students, that most listed goals involved health self-improvement. We wished to know if categories of self-improvement were cognized differently vis-à-vis their functional attributes (direction, regulation, control, and arousal). If there were notable differences, we reasoned that goal attainment might ultimately be affected (although in this study we did not assess actual goal performance).

Table 1 presents the ratings for the control and arousal functions, contrasting groups for whom weight loss and exercise were the stated objectives. As can readily be seen, the self-directive potential of exercise exceeds that of weight loss for this sample, most notably in the arousal advantage. If, as Ford (1987) posits, the arousal function permits fine-tuning of energy production and distribution for the purpose of managing unpredictable environments, then the subjects in our sample could be expected (all other *functions* being equal) to pursue exercise goals with greater efficiency than weight loss goals. Of course, as a relational model like ours would suggest, all other functions were *not* equal—but, in general, the pattern favoring exercise over weight loss held up (exercise was seen as less difficult, more controllable, and as having a greater positive impact on health than weight loss).

TABLE 1 Comparison of college student ratings of weight loss versus exercise goals

Type of functional attribute and its indicator	Weight loss/Exercise (mean ratings)
Control	
Self-reward for goal progress	6.0 vs. 5.8
Self-punishment for goal failure	7.3 vs. 6.0**
Frequency of pursuit	7.2 vs. 7.2
Arousal	
Stress	4.6 vs. 2.0*
Absorption	4.7 vs. 5.7***
Enjoyment	3.3 vs. 6.5*

Note. From Karoly, McKeeman, and Clapper (1985, November). Adapted by permission. Ns = 100 (Weight); 105 (Exercise).

*$p < .0001$, two-tailed. **$p < .001$, two-tailed. ***$p < .003$, two-tailed.

REAL-TIME DYNAMICS AND GOAL PLANNING

The study of how individuals erect relatively stable cognitive representations of their goals must be supplemented by the study of how people formulate plans of action (still a cognitive creation) to achieve their goals in the face of an ever-changing, but predictable, reality. Planning, or problem-solving, involves the building and testing of means–ends structures. Unlike the previously noted functional, structural, and ecological cognitions, which exist within working memory in a "timeless" state, the construction of a behavioral path to goal achievement must be temporally dynamic, in the sense that the steps between wanting and getting are played out as *scenarios*—movies in the head, if you will—or projections onto what cognitive scientists call a *problem space* (cf. Newell & Simon, 1972; Wilensky, 1983). For these reasons, I refer to this aspect of the theory of goal systems as *real-time dynamics.*

To employ yet another terminology, that of Anderson (1983), we can begin to approach dynamic understanding when we move from the GSI-type assessment of *declarative* goal representations (i.e., knowledge coded as a set of facts or judgments) to an assessment of *procedural* structures, or knowledge coded in the form of condition–action (if–then) rules. If we wish to understand, at the level of behavioral enactments, why goals are persistently pursued, altered, redirected, replaced, abandoned, put aside, or recharged after a period of inactivity, we should look, I believe, to the structure of people's problem-solving scenarios. Doing so might allow us to discover the coherence behind the apparent planlessness of people's lives (finding what Nesselroade and Ford [1987] called "consistencies in patterns of variability").* Goal-relevant procedural knowledge ties into Powers' (1973) cybernetic model of action control, corresponding to the concept of "program control." As Powers (1973) states:

> *The essence of a program is what computer programmers call a test, a branch-point, or an if-statement—a point where the list of questions being carried out is interrupted and some state of affairs is perceived and compared to a reference state of affairs . . . the choice points may form a network, the outcome of each test determining the path, open or closed, that will actually be followed. (p. 161)*[†]

Programs are the higher-order architects of the observable, steady-state fluctuations in day-to-day action. Programs, or if–then structures, are equivalent to Schank and Abelson's (1977) concept of *plans,* which are problem-solving routines that vary in their level of specificity. Some theorists, including Powers (1973), postulate knowledge structures at even higher levels of abstractness, including something akin to sense of self or personal *identity,* which acts as the superordinate program influencing goal-directedness through many intermediate, hierarchically-laddered levels of control (cf. Markus & Nurius, 1986; Read, 1987; Scheier & Carver, 1988; Whitbourne, 1985).

It is my contention that the planning aspect of goal systems (as a form of procedural knowledge) is an important mechanism underlying adverse health outcomes across the life span. However, rather than operating as a cognitive–structural variable, like the GSI-measured concepts previously noted or like Kobasa's (1979) notion of "hardiness," planning or problem-solving is a *process* dimension with a definite real-time trajectory. As Newell and Simon (1972) and others describe it, the process is a search through a state space consisting of an initial state, a goal state (usually several, in fact), a set of operators or behavioral enactment skills, and a set of constraints or exception rules that define the limits of acceptable action in the problem context. As noted by Holland, Holyoak, Nisbett, and Thagard (1986), the problem-solver conducts a means–ends analysis by (a) comparing goals against current states and

*Recall the automobile trip metaphor and my criticism of fuel-centered and destination-centered models. Clearly, in seeking to explain why a journey is suddenly canceled, why a side trip is added, why a stay in one spot is longer or shorter than originally planned, or why travel continues despite warnings of danger on the road ahead, neither the vehicle-centered nor the journey-centered approach will suffice. Now we must become *driver-centered.* Unlike some of my colleagues, I do not see the use of personality traits or styles as being of much assistance here. In fact, I see personality as a vehicle-centered (structural) approach, which does not address steady-state transitions in the way that self-reflective, propositional knowledge systems do.

[†]*Note.* From *Behavior: The Control of Perception* by W. T. Powers, 1973. Hawthorne, New York: Aldine Publishing Company. Copyright 1973. Reprinted by permission.

noting discrepancies; (b) selecting an operator to correct the discrepancy; (c) applying the operator if feasible and, if not, transforming the current state into one in which the operator can work; and (d) repeating the cycle until all discrepancies are eliminated (the goal is attained) or until a failure criterion (quit rule) or exception is encountered.

I submit that, in many situations, unhealthful, risky, or health-compromising actions on the part of either well or diagnosably ill persons are driven by age-specific, normative, goal-centered condition–action rules (or programs), which do not include avoidance of possible ill-health effects within their default hierarchies. Similarly, when people try to institute explicit programs for health promotion (e.g., diets, exercise programs), they often fail because of deficiencies in rule use. Colloquially put, *illness results from bad planning!*

As simplistic as this general hypotheses may seem, its potential power remains untapped. In seeking to prevent obesity, smoking, AIDS, drug addiction, teenage pregnancies, and other public health problems, I see researchers examining attitudinal antecedents, personality styles, social influence networks, and other psychosocial variables. I do not see any widespread examination of the role of normative social incentives or of the contents and operating characteristics of people's goal-centered declarative and procedural knowledge systems. Bad planning and faulty goal structuring might well emerge as accounting for significant illness variance. For further discussions of the dynamics of planning and procedures for assessing the structure of problem-solving networks, refer to Graesser and Clark (1985), Holland and others (1986), Read (1987), and Wilensky (1983).

GOAL SYSTEMS EQUALS LIFESTYLE

Farquhar (1987) referred to "lifestyle" as

> *the aggregate of genetic factors, the influence of early experiences and learning, and personal habits concerning diet, exercise, smoking, and stress. (p. 4)*

Alternatively, Steffen and Karoly (1980) defined "lifestyle" as

> *the idiosyncratic and characteristic approach that the person takes toward living in his physical and social world. (p. 16)*

Interestingly, in contemporary health psychology, which has sought to address the behavioral factors underlying mortality and morbidity risk, the assault on lifestyle change has been largely disorder-specific and context-specific, rarely addressing the aggregate of factors or the person's characteristic approach to living. Why people drink, smoke, drive recklessly, eat too much or too little, fail to take precautions or heed medical advice, or expose themselves to various forms of stress are questions addressed at the level of specific behaviors, precipitating situations, and motives.

Yet, all the risky activities and decisions health psychologists are hoping to influence are unified by their relationship, direct or indirect, to life tasks or goals. For this reason, it may benefit the field to broadly reconceptualize "lifestyle" as the emergent product of the declarative and procedural goal representations outlined in this chapter. Lifestyles reflect plans and goal structures; and the long-term therapeutic alteration of lifestyles rests upon goal systems "diagnosis" as a prerequisite to intervention.

CONCLUSION

Many readers may feel that the present chapter is premature, since the systems framework proposed has yet to be fully tested empirically. Yet, I have tried to show that the extant data on specific components are encouraging and that the model itself may help push back the frontiers of motivational process analysis applied in the context of health protection/health promotion. Goal systems theory and methods are truly new directions in health psychology as this chapter is being written. Yet, models like the one outlined on these pages are being welcomed within personality and cognitive psychology as containing fresh solutions to some old and thorny problems of description, prediction, and control. I trust that a similar fate awaits the goal systems perspective within health psychology.

REFERENCES

Aldenderfer, M. S., & Blashfield, R. K. (1984). *Cluster analysis.* Beverly Hills, CA: Sage.

Anderson, J. R. (1983). *The architecture of cognition.* Cambridge, MA: Harvard University Press.

Bandura, A. (1986). *Social foundations of thought and action: A social cognitive theory.* Englewood Cliffs, NJ: Prentice Hall.

Baumeister, R. F. (Ed.). (1986). *Public self and private self.* New York: Springer-Verlag.

Becker, M. H., & Maiman, L. A. (1975). Sociobehavioral determinants of compliance with health and medical care recommendations. *Medical Care, 13,* 10–24.

Calnan, M. W., & Moss, S. (1984). The health belief model and compliance with education given at a class in breast self-examination. *Journal of Health and Social Behavior, 25,* 198–210.

Cantor, N., Brower, A., & Korn, H. (1985). Cognitive bases of personality in a life transition. In E. E. Roskam (Ed.), *Measurement and personality assessment* (pp. 323–331). New York: Elsevier (North Holland).

Cantor, N., Markus, H., Niedenthal, P., & Nurius, P. (1986). On motivation and the self-concept. In R. M. Sorrentino & E. T. Higgins (Eds.), *Handbook of motivation and cognition* (pp. 96–121). New York: Guilford.

Carver, C. S., & Scheier, M. F. (1981). *Attention and self-regulation.* New York: Springer-Verlag.

Cleary, P. D. (1987). Why people take precautions against health risks. In N. D. Weinstein (Ed.), *Taking care* (pp. 119–149). New York: Cambridge University Press.

Cohen, S., & Wills, T. A. (1985). Stress, social support, and the buffering hypothesis. *Psychological Bulletin, 98,* 310–357.

Csikszentmihalyi, M. (1975). *Beyond boredom and anxiety.* San Francisco: Jossey-Bass.

Csikszentmihalyi, M., & Larson, R. (1984). *Being adolescent: Conflict and growth in the teenage years.* New York: Basic Books.

Diener, E., Emmons, R. A., Larsen, R. J., & Griffin, S. (1985). The Satisfaction With Life Scale. *Journal of Personality Assessment, 49,* 71–75.

Dorner, D. (1985). Thinking and the organization of action. In J. Kuhl & J. Beckmann (Eds.), *Action control: From cognition to behavior* (pp. 219–235). New York: Springer-Verlag.

Elliott, E. S., & Dweck, C. S. (1988). Goals: An approach to motivation and achievement. *Journal of Personality and Social Psychology, 54,* 5–12.

Emmons, R. A. (1986). Personal strivings: An approach to personality and subjective well-being. *Journal of Personality and Social Psychology, 51,* 1058–1068.

Emmons, R. A. (1989). The personal striving approach to personality. In L. A. Pervin (Ed.), *Goal concepts in personality and social cognition* (pp. 87–126). Hillsdale, NJ: Erlbaum.

Emmons, R. A., & King, L. A. (1988). Conflict among personal strivings: Immediate and long-term implications for psychological and physical well-being. *Journal of Personality and Social Psychology, 54,* 1040–1048.

Farquhar, J. W. (1987). *The American way of life need not be hazardous to your health* (rev. ed.). Reading, MA: Addison-Wesley.

Feather, N. T. (Ed.). (1982). *Expectations and actions: Expectancy-value models in psychology.* Hillsdale, NJ: Erlbaum.

Feuerstein, M., Labbe, E. E., & Kuczmierczyk, A. R. (1986). *Health psychology: A psychobiological perspective.* New York: Plenum.

Filsinger, E. E., & Karoly, P. (1985). Taxonomic methods in health psychology. In P. Karoly (Ed.), *Measurement strategies in health psychology* (pp. 373–400). New York: Wiley.

Fiore, J., Becker, J., & Coppel, D. B. (1983). Social network interactions: A buffer or a stress? *American Journal of Community Psychology, 11,* 423–439.

Ford, D. H. (1987). *Humans as self-constructing living systems: A developmental perspective on behavior and personality.* Hillsdale, NJ: Erlbaum.

Ford, M. E., & Nichols, C. W. (1987). A taxonomy of human goals and some possible applications. In M. E. Ford & D. H. Ford (Eds.), *Humans as self-constructing living systems: Putting the framework to work* (pp. 289–311). Hillsdale, NJ: Erlbaum.

Gentry, W. D., & Kobasa, S. C. Q. (1984). Social and psychological resources mediating stress-illness relationships in humans. In W. D. Gentry (Ed.), *Handbook of behavioral medicine* (pp. 87–116). New York: Guilford.

Graesser, A. C., & Clark, L. F. (1985). *Structures and procedures of implicit knowledge.* Norwood, NJ: Ablex Publishing.

Harris, D. M., & Guten, S. (1979). Health protective behavior: An exploratory study. *Journal of Health and Social Behavior, 20,* 17–29.

Holland, J. H., Holyoak, K. J., Nisbett, R. E., & Thagard, P. R. (1986). *Induction: Processes of inference, learning, and discovery.* Cambridge, MA: MIT Press.

Johnson-Laird, P. N. (1988). *The computer and the mind: An introduction to cognitive science.* Cambridge, MA: Harvard University Press.

Karoly, P., & Bay, R. C. (1988, August). *Diabetes self-care goals and their relation to children's metabolic control.* Paper presented at the 96th Annual Convention of the American Psychological Association, Atlanta, Georgia.

Karoly, P., McKeeman, D., & Clapper, R. L. (1985, November). *A structural analysis of weight regulation and exercise goals: General and self-regulatory dimensions of "personal projects" in a nonclinical sample.* Paper presented at the 19th Annual Convention of the Association for the Advancement of Behavior Therapy, Houston, Texas.

Klinger, E. (1975). Consequences of commitment to and disengagement from incentives. *Psychological Review, 82,* 1–25.

Kobasa, S. C. (1979). Stressful life events and health: An inquiry into hardiness. *Journal of Personality and Social Psychology, 37,* 1–11.

Krantz, D. S., & Glass, D. C. (1984). Personality, behavior patterns, and physical illness: Conceptual and methodological issues. In W. D. Gentry (Ed.), *Handbook of behavioral medicine* (pp. 38–86). New York: Guilford.

Kuhl, J. (1985). Volitional mediators of cognition–behavior consistency: Self regulatory processes and action versus state orientation. In J. Kuhl & J. Beckman (Eds.), *Action control* (pp. 101–128). New York: Springer-Verlag.

Kuhl, J., & Beckman, J. (Eds.). (1985). *Action control.* New York: Springer-Verlag.

Kuhlen, R. G. (1968). Developmental changes in motivation during the adult years. In B. L. Neugarten (Ed.), *Middle age and aging: A reader in social psychology* (pp. 115–136). Chicago: University of Chicago Press.

Kuhlen, R. G., & Johnson, G. H. (1952). Changes in goals with adult increasing age. *Journal of Consulting Psychology, 16,* 1–4.

Lazarus, R. S., & Folkman, S. (1984). *Stress, appraisal and coping.* New York: Springer.

Lin, N., Dean, A., & Ensel, W. (1986). *Social support, life events, and depression.* New York: Academic Press.

Linville, P. W. (1985). Self-complexity and affective extremity: Don't put all your eggs in one cognitive basket. *Social Cognition, 3,* 94–120.

Linville, P. W. (1987). Self-complexity as a cognitive buffer against stress-related illness and depression. *Journal of Personality and Social Psychology, 52,* 662–676.

Little, B. (1983). Personal projects: A rationale and method for investigation. *Environment and Behavior, 15,* 273–309.

Little, B. R. (1987a). Personal projects analysis: A new methodology for counselling psychology. *Natcon, 13,* 591–614.

Little, B. R. (1987b). Personal projects and fuzzy selves: Aspects of self-identity in adolescence. In T. Honess & K. Yardley (Eds.), *Self and identity: Perspectives across the life span* (pp. 230–245). New York: Routledge & Kegan Paul.

Lockard, J. S., & Paulus, D. L. (Eds.). (1988). *Self-deception: An adaptive mechanism?* Englewood Cliffs, NJ: Prentice Hall.

Locke, E. A., Shaw, K. N., Saari, L. M., & Latham, G. P. (1981). Goal setting and task performance: 1969–1980. *Psychological Bulletin, 90,* 125–152.

Manning, M. M., & Wright, T. L. (1983). Self-efficacy expectancies, outcome expectancies, and the persistence of pain control in childbirth. *Journal of Personality and Social Psychology, 45,* 421–431.

Markus, H., & Nurius, P. (1986). Possible selves. *American Psychologist, 41,* 954–969.

Marlatt, G. A. (1985). Cognitive factors in the relapse process. In G. A. Marlatt & J. R. Gordon (Eds.), *Relapse prevention* (pp. 128–200). New York: Guilford.

Matarazzo, J. D., Weiss, S. M., Herd, J. A., Miller, N. E., & Weiss, S. M. (Eds.). (1984). *Behavioral health: A handbook of health enhancement and disease prevention.* New York: Wiley.

Miller, G., Galanter, E., & Pribram, K. (1960). *Plans and the structure of behavior.* New York: Holt.

Nesselroade, J. R., & Ford, D. H. (1987). Methodological considerations in modeling living systems. In M. E. Ford & D. H. Ford (Eds.), *Humans as self-constructing living systems: Putting the framework to work* (pp. 47–79). Hillsdale, NJ: Erlbaum.

Newell, A., & Simon, H. A. (1972). *Human problem solving*. Englewood Cliffs, NJ: Prentice Hall.

Nuttin, J. (19840. *Motivation, planning and action: A relational theory of behavior dynamics*. Hillsdale, NJ: Erlbaum.

O'Leary, A. (1985). Self-efficacy and health. *Behavior Research and Therapy, 23,* 437–451.

Palys, T. S., & Little, B. R. (1983). Perceived life satisfaction and the organization of personal project systems. *Journal of Personality and Social Psychology, 44,* 1221–1230.

Pervin, L. A. (1983). The stasis and flow of behavior: Toward a theory of goals. In M. M. Page (Ed.), *Nebraska Symposium on Motivation* (pp. 1–53). Lincoln, NE: University of Nebraska Press.

Powers, W. T. (1973). *Behavior: The control of perception.* Chicago: Aldine.

Pyszczynski, T., & Greenberg, J. (1987). Self-regulatory perseveration and the depressive self-focusing style: A self-awareness theory of reactive depression. *Psychological Bulletin, 102,* 122–138.

Read, S. J. (1987). Constructing causal scenarios: A knowledge structure approach to causal reasoning. *Journal of Personality and Social Psychology, 52,* 288–302.

Rook, K. S. (1984). The negative side of social interaction: Impact on psychological well-being. *Journal of Personality and Social Psychology, 46,* 1097–1108.

Roskies, E. (1980). Considerations in developing a treatment program for the coronary-prone (Type A) behavior pattern. In P. O. Davidson & S. M. Davidson (Eds.), *Behavioral medicine: Changing health lifestyles* (pp. 299–333). New York: Brunner/Mazel.

Ruehlman, L. S., & Wolchik, S. A. (1988). Personal goals and interpersonal support and hindrance as factors in psychological distress and well-being. *Journal of Personality and Social Psychology, 55,* 293–301.

Sarason, I. G., & Sarason, B. R. (1985). *Social support: Theory, research, and applications.* Dordrecht: Martinus Nijhoff.

Schank, R. C., & Abelson, R. (1977). *Scripts, plans, goals, and understanding.* Hillsdale, NJ: Erlbaum.

Scheier, M. F., & Carver, C. S. (1985). Optimism, coping, and health: Assessment and implications of generalized outcome expectancies. *Health Psychology, 4,* 219–247.

Scheier, M. F., & Carver, C. S. (1988). A model of behavioral self-regulation: Translating intention into action. In L. Berkowitz (Ed.), *Advances in experimental social psychology* (Vol. 21, pp. 303–346). New York: Academic Press.

Scheier, M. F., Weintraub, J. K., & Carver, C. S. (1986). Coping with stress: Divergent strategies of optimists and pessimists. *Journal of Personality and Social Psychology, 51,* 1257–1264.

Scott, W., Osgood, D. W., & Peterson, C. (1979). *Cognitive structure.* Washington, DC: Winston & Sons.

Shumaker, S. A., & Grunberg, N. E. (1986). Proceedings of the National Working Conference on Smoking Relapse. *Health Psychology, 5*(Suppl.), 1–99.

Steffen, J. J., & Karoly, P. (1980). Toward a psychology of therapeutic persistence. In P. Karoly & J. J. Steffen (Eds.), *Improving the long-term effects of psychotherapy* (pp. 3–24). New York: Gardner Press.

Taylor, S. E. (1986). *Health psychology.* New York: Random House.

Veroff, J., & Veroff, J. B. (1980). *Social incentives: A life-span developmental approach.* New York: Academic Press.

Viet, C. T., & Ware, J. E., Jr. (1983). The structure of psychological distress and well-being in general populations. *Journal of Consulting and Clinical Psychology, 51,* 730–742.

Wadsworth, M. W., & Ford, D. H. (1983). Assessment of personal goal hierarchies. *Journal of Counseling Psychology, 30,* 514–526.

Wallston, B. S., Alagna, S. W., DeVellis, B. M., & DeVellis, R. F. (1983). Social support and physical health. *Health Psychology, 2,* 367–391.

Watson, D. (1988). Intraindividual and interindividual analyses of positive and negative affect: Their relation to health complaints, perceived stress, and daily activities. *Journal of Personality and Social Psychology, 54,* 1020–1030.

Watson, D., & Clark, L. A. (1984). Negative affectivity: The disposition to experience aversive emotional states. *Psychological Bulletin, 96,* 465–490.

Watson, D., Clark, L. A., & Tellegen, A. (1988). Development and validation of brief measures of positive and negative affect: The PANAS scales. *Journal of Personality and Social Psychology, 54,* 1063–1070.

Watson, D., & Tellegen, A. (1985). Toward a consensual structure of mood. *Psychological Bulletin, 98,* 219–235.

Weinstein, N. D. (Ed.). (1987). *Taking care: Understanding and encouraging self-protective behavior.* New York: Cambridge University Press.

Weinstein, N. D. (1988). The precaution adoption process. *Health Psychology, 7,* 355–386.

Whitbourne, S. K. (1985). The psychological construction of the life span. In J. E. Birren & K. W. Schaie (Eds.), *Handbook of the psychology of aging.* New York: Van Nostrand.

Wicklund, R. A., & Gollwitzer, P. M. (1982). *Symbolic self-completion.* Hillsdale, NJ: Erlbaum.

Wilensky, R. (1983). *Planning and understanding*. Reading, MA: Addison-Wesley.

Winell, M. (1987). Personal goals: The key to self-direction in adulthood. In M. E. Ford & D. H. Ford (Eds.), *Humans as self-constructing living systems: Putting the framework to work* (pp. 261–287). Hillsdale, NJ: Erlbaum.

4

ASSESSING HEALTH RISKS IN THE WORK SETTING

Stanislav V. Kasl

Yale University School of Medicine

INTRODUCTION

This chapter has several objectives, which come together in the somewhat unwieldy question: What aspects or dimensions of the work environment should we measure, why should we be concerned with them, and how should they be measured? In other words, I wish to consider the empirical evidence about the impact of the work environment on health, while also dealing with specific issues of measurement. In addition, I wish to provide a forward-looking perspective so that I can raise issues about what we should know, rather than be bound by narrow summaries of what we do know (or seem to know) already.

The material relevant for this chapter comes from diverse sources—diverse disciplines, methodologies, and research topics. In some sense, I shall be trying to integrate the perspectives of occupational and psychosocial epidemiology, behavioral medicine, health psychology, psychosomatic medicine, medical sociology, and social and organizational psychology. Because of the near-impossibility of integrating such a diversity of perspectives, I have chosen epidemiology to provide for me the primary framework for examining issues of methodology and evidence.

A traditional chapter dealing with measurement or assessment tends to be organized around classical issues of reliability and validity, pertaining to measures of distinct concepts or dimensions. The recitation of studies showing adequate reliability (mostly coefficient alpha) tends to be impressive, but the review of validity gets easily bogged down in uncertainties regarding just what kinds of data should be viewed as evidence of validity and how inadequate the cumulative evidence actually is. A good traditional chapter may then return to broader issues of theory and conceptualization and offer some suggestions for revisions or refinements.

In the present chapter I do not wish to follow such an approach. There are several reasons for this: (a) Traditional psychometric notions of reliability and validity come to us from studies of traits and abilities, while I wish to concentrate on environmental variables for which such notions may have only selected applicability. For example, if the dimension of "machine-paced work" has significance for the health of blue-collar workers (e.g., Smith, 1985), then psychometric questions about reliability and validity may not be the best strategy for probing into the general issue of how to best measure the exposure to such a work condition. (b) In the traditional approach, the link between the conceptualization of a construct and its actual operationalization determines in large part what type of empirical evidence is to be viewed as relevant for validity, particularly construct validity. In the present chapter, however, the emphasis is on evidence regarding the impact on health, whether or not such evidence should be interpreted as contributing to the construct validity of a measure or an assessment procedure. Furthermore, suggestions regarding changes in measurement procedures will be offered from the perspective of improving our ability to detect health impact and not from any concern for narrowing a possible discrepancy between conceptualization and operationalization. Clearly then, the emphasis on health impact, while appropriate to the stated objectives of this chapter, would normally be too narrow and too off-target in the usual psychology-oriented review of measurement procedures. (c) I intend to place the consideration of the issue of measurement in the context of a broader examination of adequacy of research methodology for detecting health impact. I believe there are four components which come together in an adequate methodology:

1. the adequacy of the design of the study, which in the typical quasi-experimental research means what data are collected from (or about) what subjects at what time;
2. the adequacy of the conceptualization and operationalization of the exposure or risk factors;
3. the adequacy of data analysis, both from the perspective of ruling out alternate explanations as well as the perspective of testing a particular causal or conceptual model; and
4. the adequacy of the theoretical formulation regarding the etiological dynamics of the exposure–disease outcome process.

AN EPIDEMIOLOGICAL PERSPECTIVE ON WORK AND HEALTH

The choice of an epidemiological perspective as the framework for examining issues of methodology and evidence is based, in part, on my experience in attempting to evaluate the work and health evidence and to come to grips with various research design and measurement problems (e.g., Kasl, 1978, 1985, 1986). However, a more important consideration for choosing the epidemiological approach is the subject matter itself: (a) The primary risk factors (independent variables) of interest are dimensions of the environment, not personality traits or social perceptions and attitudes; and (b) the primary outcomes of interest are health/illness, defined with the help of biomedical parameters, not feelings or behavior. In other words, the anchor points of our methodological and substantive exploration are, on the one hand, environmental conditions that are susceptible to objective definition and measurement (i.e., not involving an individual's cognitive and emotional processing; see Frese & Zapf, 1988) and on the other hand, disease states/illness, physical disability, subclinical disease, symptoms, and elevated biomedical risk factors. The discipline most appropriate for studying the causal link between these two anchors is epidemiology. The social and behavioral sciences have a vital contribution to make in elaborating on and enriching our understanding of the processes involved, in directing our attention to particular aspects of the work setting, and in helping us formulate conceptual and research strategies that are most sensitive for detecting health impact. But we cannot give up on the notions that the environment is more than psychological perceptions and appraisals ("the environment which is in the head"); the mediating processes are biological as well as psychosocial; and the outcomes are biomedical, not just behavioral and affective.

The basics of the epidemiological perspective can be restated as follows: Our primary goal is to identify linkages between exposure to some aspect of the (objective) work environment and adverse (or, possibly, positive) health outcomes. We should design our studies and conduct our analyses so as to optimize our chances of demonstrating that such linkages in fact represent cause–effect relationships. Additional effort that goes into designing the study, such as additional data collection or data analysis, should be in the service of the primary goal (e.g., eliminating self-selection biases) or of two additional goals: (a) to identify variables that explain additional variance in the adverse health outcomes and, thereby, indicate differential reactivity to the environmental exposure and (b) to provide information to the underlying mechanisms involved in the overall association. Obviously, the two additional goals are well intertwined; advancing one is likely to advance the other.

It is useful to outline the elements of our ideal study design in occupational (psychosocial) epidemiology—not because we will be able to implement it with any great frequency in our actual work, but because the listing of its components alerts us to possible design weaknesses when one or more are absent. The fundamental design is what I have called elsewhere (Kasl, 1983) a "doubly prospective" one: The cohort is enrolled in the study before the development of the disease outcome of interest *and* before the exposure of interest. Other elements in this strong design may be listed as follows:

1. The environmental condition (exposure) is objectively defined and measured.
2. Self-selection into exposure conditions is minimized by exploiting opportunities for "natural experiments," changes in the work setting that lead to highly comparable groups of exposed and unexposed individuals.
3. Potential confounding variables, such as biological risk factors, are assessed and their influence monitored in analysis.
4. The period of follow-up is adequate both for the purpose of seeing the cohort through the stages of impact and adaptation to the environmental exposure (if there are, in fact, any such stages) and through the full etiological sequence of disease development.
5. Mediating processes are studied and vulnerability factors that interact with exposure are included.

In actual practice, the designs that have provided information on work and health understandably fall short of this ideal in one or more respects. One quite reasonable approximation of the above ideal is the historical cohort study: On the basis of past records one reconstructs a cohort as it existed at some point in the past and "follows" it forward into the present through historical data which provide information on past occupational exposures and disease outcomes. Certain conditions should hold for this to be an effective design: (a) The reconstructed cohort represents a meaningful and generalizable group of subjects; (b) the historical starting point is appropriate for the task of detecting the disease impact of exposure, since it takes the cohort through the full etiological sequence of disease development; (c) there is a complete monitoring of the cohort to determine later exposures, disease onset, and various attrition pathways (e.g., death, retirement, transfer, geographical move); and (d) there is a sufficiently powerful statistical technique applied to the data, such as survival analysis with time-dependent and time-independent covariants. Common limitations of the approach are loss to follow-up, incomplete or biased ascertainment of cases of disease, inaccurate (or incomplete or insufficiently relevant) exposure data, and inability to add to the original pool of available information except through retrospection from an attrition-biased set of "survivors." It should be emphasized that the historical cohort design is not the same as simply starting out with a cross-sectional sample and obtaining on them, from records, historical information; the latter design may not enable us to reconstruct the original cohort from which the present sample is an undetermined subset.

There is another design, which often looks a bit better than it is: A sample of subjects, often beautifully representative, is targeted for longitudinal data collection. I have referred to this as a "slice of life" longitudinal design (Kasl, 1983). Even when the variables, chosen for repeated data collection, are thoughtfully selected, there may still be a problem with the arbitrary window of observation we will have on each individual. In effect, our subjects will be at different stages of the exposure–adaptation–impact etiological dynamics; some will be observed too early, others too late, and combining the information for the total sample as if Time 1, Time 2, and so on had the same meaning and temporal location for all individuals cannot but dilute our power to detect the etiological processes. In studies of acute events (such as bereavement or retirement), we are beginning to recognize the need to coordinate the scheduling of the data collection to the temporal aspects of the event. But in the case of chronic exposures, such as to the work setting, we have apparently convinced ourselves that just when we start our observation on an individual and when we complete it is not really important for detecting the impact of the exposure. It might be noted that the statistical procedure of treating Time 1 data as covariants for Time 2 (or later) data does not alleviate this problem, but is rather a formal expression of it: Just as the "window of observation" means we don't know what went on before (and after), so too the Time 1 covariants are meant to adjust out prior impact.

An actual example may illustrate this point better. There is considerable evidence from the mental health literature on blue-collar workers in assembly-line jobs (e.g., Caplan, Cobb, French, Harrison, & Pinneau, 1975; Chinoy, 1955; Kasl, 1974; Kornhauser, 1965) that adaptation to a boring, monotonous job takes place rather early in their careers, that the primary mode of adaptation is giving up on expecting work to be a meaningful human activity, and that those unable to adapt "successfully" are likely to drift out of such jobs. Under these circumstances, a beautiful 5-year longitudinal study of blue-collar workers of a wide age range might miss the boat altogether on reconstructing properly the dynamics of impact of assembly line work.

In addition to the historical cohort and the "slice of life" longitudinal approach, occupational epidemiology offers many studies using some form of a cross-sectional design. At its best, this involves a well-defined representative sample and appropriate assessments of occupational exposures and health status (prevalent disease). At its worst, we may be looking at a case-control design in which the cases of disease are an unknown subset of all persons with the disease, due to unsystematic and/or haphazard and/or biased enrollment of cases into the study; the controls are of dubious comparability; and exposure data are purely subjective and retrospective. A recent report using national Health Examination Survey data (Karasek et al., 1988) is an illustration of a strong cross-sectional study: A national sample of employed males is used to describe the association between a specific occupational characteristic (high psychological work load together with low decision latitude, using an imputation procedure to classify census occupations) and prevalence of myocardial infarction (MI). Of course, the inherent limitations of this design cannot be overcome by the presence of good sampling and strong measurements. We are dealing with survivors, and any association of case fatality rates with occupational variables could distort the cross-sectional data. Also, risk factors measured after the disease may not be an accurate characterization of their levels before disease. In fact, in the multivariable logistic regression analysis carried out by Karasek and others (1988), systolic blood pressure had a small negative association with MI. In view of ample prospective data on the role of high blood pressure in MI (Pooling Project Research Group, 1978), we know not to trust this awkward negative association in the cross-sectional data; unfortunately, we don't have similar rich prospective data on work conditions and MI to guide our interpretations.

In this section on the epidemiological perspective, I have outlined an orientation and discussed selected research design issues. The orientation fundamentally cautions against the practice of translating the primary independent, process, and dependent variables into purely psychological concepts and psychological measurements: Subjective measures of exposure replace objective approaches to environmental conditions, phenomenological reconstructions of cognitive processes replace the study of biological pathways, and indicators of distress and dissatisfaction act as proxies for health outcomes. Since this orientation may seem unduly prescriptive and proscriptive, and insufficiently appreciative of the contribution of the social and behavioral sciences, I wish to restate my orientation in a somewhat different way (and to justify it by examples in later sections of this chapter).

Clearly, investigators are not obliged to defend the choice of their subject matter or to accept some reductionistic hierarchical schema of the sciences where biomedical approaches are somehow seen as more fundamental than social and psychological approaches. However, investigators should state clearly what they intend to study, and they should understand what research designs go best with what objectives. Consider the subjective appraisal of "my job is demanding" as the focal concept. Our objectives can be to study (a) the health consequences of such appraisal, (b) the antecedents in the work environment, (c) the phenomenological/cognitive antecedents, (d) the psychological/behavioral consequence, and (e) the mediating and/or moderating role of such appraisal in the environmental exposure and health outcome association. Other combinations and refinements of these objectives are, of course, possible. The points to remember are that these objectives are distinct and should not be confused with each other or with other objectives because they do not provide interchangeable information, and that the designs actually used may or may not permit the use of such strongly inferential terminology as "antecedents" and "consequences."

DIMENSIONALIZING THE WORK ENVIRONMENT

If one reflects on the central question posed in the introduction, the task for this chapter becomes quite daunting. One major issue is, how does one go about dimensionalizing the work environment and/or developing an adequate taxonomy? One possible way to go is to pretend we are dealing with personality traits and to mimic the procedure that Cattell (1957) utilized when he set out to map the total domain of personality: We use a dictionary to develop a large list of descriptive words and phrases pertaining to the work environment, prune the list by removing synonyms and redundancies, and then develop individual scale items. We thus generate a large pool, which we can then subject to some dimensional analysis, such as factor analysis. This procedure appears systematic and comprehensive, but it does run into several difficulties. One concern is that our language (and therefore our dictionaries) is more attuned to describing people than the work environment, which may include new and unique physical characteristics or man–machine interactions. This would make the procedure more suitable for dimensionalizing personality than for dimensionalizing the work environment. Another difficulty concerns the decision to whom to administer the pool of items: To job occupants or to "observers" rating jobs? And how in the analysis do we pay attention to within-jobs and across-jobs information?

Another serious problem is that the whole procedure begs the question of what is the generic meaning of "work environment?" Thus, which aspects of the physical environment should be included and which ones excluded? One might, for example, exclude radon gas concentrations on the grounds that the causal pathway to increased risk to lung cancer does not involve psychological variables, but one would include occupational noise because it appears richly linked to psychosocial variables (Evans, 1982; Jones & Chapman, 1984). But this distinction is fuzzy at best, and is dependent on current knowledge; thus, for example, we have recently learned that specific ergonomic factors (i.e., the adequacy of back support provided by the chair in which a VDT operator sits) may interact with the dimension of low control to produce a variety of stress-related symptoms (Haynes, LaCroix, & Lippin, 1987).

The domain of work environment dimensions is also ambiguous because we don't know if we are trying to include isolated environmental descriptors, or more complex transactional terms reflecting the man–machine interaction and the person–environment fit. For example, in characterizing one aspect of job demands of a particular secretarial job, we could restrict ourselves to the expectation (demand) of typing at an average rate of eight error-free manuscript pages per hour, or we could characterize this job demand by a more complex combination of demand, equipment available, and typing skills of the individual. A similar issue involves the whole domain of "nonwork roles" (e.g., Gutek, Repetti, & Silver, 1988), which may provide important context for specific work environmental dimensions, such as job demands, thus altering their meaning and, eventually, their impact. For example, the limited benefits of flextime on absenteeism and possibly job satisfaction may hold primarily for women who have primary responsibility for small children (e.g., Hicks & Klimoski, 1981; Krausz & Freibach, 1983; Narayanan & Nath, 1982). These are difficult questions and the current popularity of complex relational terms, such as Person–Environment Fit (e.g., French, Caplan, & Van Harrison, 1982) and stress as excess of environmental demands over the individual's capacity to meet them (e.g., McGrath, 1970) invites the creation of complex variables which package together stimulus and response characteristics or stimulus and context variables. But the optimal strategy would still seem to be to develop measures of unidimensional characteristics of only the work environment and to treat all complex relational or transactional formulations as invitations to test interactive relationships at the stage of data analysis.

The question may be raised whether a detailed listing of all occupations, such as a dictionary of occupational titles (U.S. Department of Commerce, 1980) might serve as a starting point for dimensionalizing the work environment or developing a taxonomy. The answer would seem to be "with difficulty." What would be the basis on which we could take such a large set of nominal categories and create meaningful clusters, and then derive, from such a clustering, specific dimensions? Basically, we would need to have the list of dimensions (for which we are searching) already, as well as the scores on these dimensions for each job, if we were to develop a basis for clustering the occupations. It is possible that a large number of expert judges could be asked to make judgments of similarity (proximity) of occupations, according to some suitable psychophysical procedure for obtaining judgments. Multidimensional techniques would then be applied to these proximity or similarity judgments. Since the dimensions thus generated would be defined by actual occupational titles, one would still need to make inferences (interpretations) regarding the underlying work environmental dimensions. And it is doubtful that expert judges sufficiently familiar with such a spectrum of occupations could actually be found.

It would appear to be reasonable to conclude that (a) no systematic effort to dimensionalize the work environment has been undertaken, and (b) the proper empirical procedures for pursuing such a goal are difficult to formulate. This state of affairs is not unusual, since related domains of inquiry are in a similar position. For example, with respect to the residential environment, very little has been done toward developing systematically an adequate set of dimensions. Perhaps the most ambitious and best thought-through classification schema of properties of the built environment, relevant to behavior and health, was offered by Geddes and Gutman (1977). The classification schema consist of 48 categories of environments, based on the conjunction of six levels of environmental scale (e.g., building, site plan, neighborhood layout) and eight "properties'' of environments (e.g., spatial organization, amenities, architectonic properties). Such a schema suggests a formidable complexity, since within each of the 48 categories, specific environmental dimensions still have to be identified. The potential that a similar complexity would apply to dimensionalizing the work environment is very high.

Given the absence of a comprehensive and systematic effort to dimensionalize the work environment, we need to be pragmatic about discussing this issue of dimensions of the work environment. One approach is to examine some influential studies. One such study is *Job Demands and Worker Health* (Caplan et al., 1975), a cross-sectional survey of some 23 occupational groups derived from 67 different sites or organizational affiliations. The study was conducted at the Institute for Social Research (ISR), University of Michigan, and included measures which had been developed at ISR during the previous 15 years of research, including such classics as *Organizational Stress: Studies in Role Conflict and Ambiguity* (Kahn, Wolfe, Quinn, Snoek, & Rosenthal, 1964). The self-report measures of the work environment included hours worked per week, hours of overtime, unwanted overtime, quantitative work load, variance in work load, responsibility for persons, job complexity, concentration, role conflict, role ambiguity, job future ambiguity, underutilization of abilities, inequity of pay, participation, and social support from supervisor and from others at work. The study also included several measures of ''personal preferences'' with respect to the work environment: quantitative work load, responsibility for persons, job complexity, and role ambiguity. This permitted the construction of four person–environment (P–E) fit measures. The results with these P–E fit measures were reported in detail in a later volume (French et al., 1982).

Another influential source of measures are the two national surveys conducted by ISR for the U.S. Department of Labor (Quinn et al., 1971; Quinn & Sheppard, 1974). An important purpose in those surveys was to assess the frequency and severity of work-related problems experienced by employed people. Among the relevant measures utilized in these surveys were the following: (a) An index of labor standards problem areas involving inquiry into 19 areas, among them health and safety hazards, transportation problems, fringe benefits, work hours, unsteady employment, invasion of privacy, problems with union, and age and/or sex discrimination. The level of detail in assessing these varied considerably; thus, for example, the ''health and safety hazards'' was one of the richer scales and included about 20 different items. (b) A number of measures reflecting ''context of work,'' including ease of changing job assignment, demand characteristics of job, autonomy and control, time pressures, resource adequacy, and utilization of education and skills. (c) Other measures of possible interest included dimensions of supervisory behavior, interpersonal relations, and meaning of work (different functions it served for the worker).

Another pragmatic source of dimensions of work environment are job satisfaction studies. The literature is, of course, enormous but does show a fair amount of consistency or convergence. At minimum the literature illustrates what dimensions are considered important by investigators focusing on one domain of impact of work. But to the extent that often large pools of job satisfaction items are subjected to some dimensional analysis, such as factor analysis (which is rarely done with the a priori scales noted above), then we in fact have some empirical basis for talking about a comprehensive set of dimensions for the work environment. (Of course, if investigators never write job satisfaction items for a particular domain of work, it will never show up as a factor in factor analysis).

The following is a listing of illustrative instruments and the dimensions which they include:

1. Minnesota Satisfaction Questionnaire (Weiss, Davis, England, & Lofquist, 1967): ability utilization, achievement, activity, advancement, authority, company policies and practices, compensation, co-workers, creativity, independence, moral values, recognition, responsibility, security, social service, social status, supervision (human relations), supervision (technical), variety, and working conditions.
2. Job Descriptive Index (Smith, Kendall, & Hulin, 1969): work itself, pay, opportunities for promotion, supervision, and co-workers.
3. Job Diagnostic Survey (Hackman & Oldham, 1975): pay, job security, social, supervisory, growth.
4. Quality of Employment Survey (Quinn & Shepard, 1974): comfort, challenge, financial rewards, relations with co-workers, resource adequacy, and promotion.
5. Index of Organizational Reactions (Smith, 1976): supervision, company identification, physical environment, financial rewards, kind of work, amount of work, co-workers, and career future.

A nice overview of the job satisfaction literature is provided by Locke (1976). A useful compilation of job satisfaction measures is provided in a recent technical report to the National Institute for Occupational Safety and Health (NIOSH) (Jenkins, DeFrank, & Speers, 1984). An earlier overview of job satisfaction measures is provided by Robinson, Athanasiou, and Head (1969).

Another perspective on work dimensions is provided by investigators who use standardized descriptions by "expert" observers who are not themselves subjects in the study (e.g., Hackman & Oldham, 1975; House, 1980; Jenkins, Nadler, Lawler, & Cammann, 1975). Two examples are (a) the Job Diagnostic Survey (Hackman & Oldham, 1975), which looks at skill variety, task identity, task significance, autonomy, feedback from the job itself, feedback from agents, and dealing with others and (b) the "Standardized Observations" approach (Jenkins et al., 1975), which focuses on variety, autonomy, external feedback, task feedback, rigidity, certainty, conflicting demands, interruptions, required skills and abilities, worker pace control, required interdependence, required cooperation, work pressures, employee effort, meaningfulness, resource adequacy, comfort, and task identity.

It may be noted that it is highly desirable to utilize sources of data about the work environment which go beyond self-reports of the respondents, who also provide information about themselves with respect to indictors of impact. At the same time, however, the use of the "expert" observers represents a missed opportunity. Fundamentally, the observers are working with the same broad subjective dimensions of the work setting as are used in the self-report scales. An optimal use of expert observers would concentrate on dimensions which are not easily accessible to normal observations (or self-observations) of the workers themselves and would emphasize technical information about the various aspects of the job, or would represent an expert interpretation of numerical data coming from instruments and tests. An analogy from the medical care setting may help here. We may collect self-report data from the patient on the likelihood that he has high blood pressure. We do not then turn around and ask the nurse for her judgment of the likelihood that the patient has high blood pressure; rather, we want her to get an actual blood pressure reading. What we need in the work and health area is a broader integration of the physical environment into our social–psychological formulations, a long-standing problem and issue for psychology (e.g., Kates and Wohlwill, 1966). We need a greater appreciation of the biobehavioral approach to the workplace (e.g., Brady & Fischman, 1986); a greater attempt to bring in other disciplines such as ergonomics (e.g., Shephard, 1974); a closer attention to classical issues in occupational medicine (e.g., Levy & Wegman, 1983; Stellman & Snow, 1986); and a greater sensitivity to specific changes taking place in the work setting, such as automation in offices (Office of Technology Assessment, 1985). It should be added that these suggestions and criticisms are much more directed to the U.S. research literature on work and health and much less so to the Scandinavian studies in the same area.

The work dimensions that have been pragmatically derived from the various sources invite several comments. A major point, already noted, is that we lack a systematic and comprehensive framework for asking whether any list of dimensions is complete or adequate, and if it is rationally organized into proper categories (e.g., mutually exclusive), hierarchically organized subcategories, and so on. Several issues are contingent on this point. One such issue is completeness. For example, an investigator with an organizational perspective (e.g., Beehr & Bhagat, 1985; Dunnette, 1976; Miles, 1980; Sethi & Schuler, 1984) would argue that important dimensions have been omitted, such as organizational size, organizational structure ("flat" vs. "tall"), staff versus line position, working on the periphery of an organization, and so on. Another issue is proper classification. For example, if one creates major categories, such as "work itself," "interpersonal aspects," "health and safety hazards," and so on, then should we consider role ambiguity as "work itself" or as "interpersonal"? A third issue is reasons for inclusion. For example, it is possible to argue that most of our dimensions of work environment are based on our notions about people (such as dimensions of needs and abilities), and we dimensionalize the work setting according to our a priori notions about people. This may not be an adequate approach, particularly if some human needs and abilities are not inherent in human nature, but rather derive out of interactions with important settings, such as work.

Another important comment that needs to be made about the pragmatic list of dimensions that tend to dominate the studies of work and health is that the formulations of these dimensions, and therefore the measurement itself, is driven by the desire to evolve universal dimensions, in the sense that they are applicable to more or less any sample of employed individuals. The advantages are obvious: We do not need to develop a plethora of specific measures, we are able to make comparisons across occupations, and we can combine respondents from different settings. But what are the disadvantages? Logically, it would seem that we are unable to study the impact of those unique aspects of work which characterize only some jobs and are not represented in these all-purpose scales. Alternately, if the important but unique work characteristics are only obliquely represented in these broad measures, then we dilute our ability to detect impact and perhaps increase the chances of incorrect interpretation of what the pathogenic exposure really is. Aside from this, I also believe that the apparent (real?) need (convenience?) for having universal or all-purpose work dimensions reinforces—and is reinforced by—the tendency toward the excessive psychologizing of our formulations and our techniques of measurement. Paying close attention to the physical work environment, to objectively defined work tasks, or to measures of task demands dependent on ergonomic or physical fitness factors, leads perforce to the abandonment of self-reports, to the need for the research team to enter the various specific work settings, and to the fractionation of measures (noncomparability across sites). Conversely, the goal of developing universal measures easily leads to formulations which drift toward the more global, the more cognitive/subjective/psychological, and away from environmental and biobehavioral.

It is, of course, incorrect to leave the impression that investigators only work with measures that are broad and cut across many occupations. Specific scales have been developed for such groups as policemen (Cooper, Davidson, & Robinson, 1982; Davidson & Veno, 1980), air traffic controllers (Crump, 1979; Rose, Jenkins, & Hurst, 1978), nurses (Gentry & Parkes, 1982; Gray-Toft & Anderson, 1981), medical technologists (Matteson & Ivancevich, 1982), teachers (Fimian, 1984; Phillis & Lee, 1980), and scientists in organizations (Pelz & Andrews, 1966). Investigators working in specific occupational settings need to consider carefully the objectives of the study: Broader measures allow comparisons with other studies conducted in different settings, while specific measures are likely to be more suitable to the dynamics of the targeted work setting.

DIMENSIONS OF THE WORK SETTING THAT ARE LIKELY TO IMPACT ON HEALTH

In this section, I wish to discuss the dimensions or aspects of the work setting that are worthy of our attention because of their probable impact on health. Since the relevant studies are so numerous, an integrated overview is very difficult. I will use a three-layered approach. First, I will pay attention to the broad literature, which deals with a variety of outcomes (e.g., job satisfaction, psychological strain, and specific diseases) and may reflect a particular orientation, most often a stress perspective. In the second step, I will try to zero in on the evidence that is specifically concerned with physical health outcomes. In the third step, I will take one particular area—control and health—in order to make my comments more concrete and precise. The emphasis throughout is on constructs and assessment.

The following reviews, overviews, and edited volumes provide a useful entree into the relevant literature: Baker, 1985; Beehr and Newman, 1978; Burke, 1984; Cataldo and Coates, 1986; Cohen and Syme, 1985; Cooper and Marshall, 1980; Cooper and Payne, 1978, 1980, 1988; Cooper and Smith, 1985; Elliott and Eisdorfer, 1982; Gardell, 1976, 1982a; Holt, 1982; House, 1980, 1981; House and Cottington, 1986; Hurrell and Colligan, 1982; Jick and Burke, 1982; Kahn, 1981; Kahn, Hein, House, Kasl, and McLean, 1982; Kasl, 1978, 1984, 1986; Kasl and Cobb, 1983; McGrath, 1976; McLean, 1979; Quick, Bhagat, Dalton, and Quick, 1987; Salvendy and Smith, 1981; Sauter, Hurrell, and Cooper, 1989; Sharit and Salvendy, 1982; Shostak, 1980; Steptoe and Mathews, 1984; Tasto, Colligan, Skjei, and Polly, 1978.

The 1976 *Handbook of Industrial and Organization Psychology* (Dunnette, 1976) has a chapter on job satisfaction by Locke (1976). On the basis of his review of the influences on job satisfaction, Locke characterized desirable conditions at work as follows: (a) Work represents mental challenge (with which the worker can cope successfully) and leads to involvement and personal interest; (b) work is not physically too tiring; (c) rewards for performance are just, informative, and in line with aspirations; (d) working conditions are compatible with physical needs and they facilitate work goals; (e) work leads to high self-esteem; and (f) agents in the workplace help with the attainment of job values. This represents an admirable summary with much intuitive appeal. For our purpose here, however, we need to remind ourselves that it is a creative summary of job satisfaction, not health impact.

In a chapter that provides an overview of the field, as well as an epilogue to the 1985 Conference on Work Stress and the Role of Health Care Delivery Systems (Quick et al., 1987), Robert Kahn (1987) offers the following classification of aspects of the work environment likely to impact on health: (a) Work deprivation (job loss, job insecurity), (b) occupation, (c) properties of the work itself (intrinsic), (d) role characteristics, (e) interpersonal relations, (f) lack of resources and equipment, (g) work schedules, and (h) organizational climate. Holt (1982) also provides a careful and systematic listing of occupational stressors that have been studied.

An integrative summary of this large and somewhat intractable literature suggests the following dimensions of the work setting which are likely to impact on health:

1. *Physical (hygienic) conditions at work:* Those related to comfort, such as heat, cold, humidity; hazardous exposures to radiation, chemical, or pollutants; other exposures that relate to symptoms or annoyance, such as dust and fumes; noise; dangerous machinery. The presumption with this list is that aside from "direct" effects (which presumably bypass cognitive or emotional processing, such as the radiation-to-cancer association), indirect effects are likely, either because awareness of exposure to hazards may have its own consequences (e.g., Kasl, Chisholm, & Eskenazi, 1981) or the physical conditions interact with psychosocial variables.
2. *Physical aspects of work:* Bad ergonomic or man–machine design; physical constraints on movement; comfort; vibrations; physical demands (e.g., lifting); and pacing by machinery, including breakdown of machinery. Clearly it is somewhat arbitrary to list these separately from the previous category above.
3. *Temporal aspects of work day and work itself:* Shift work, particularly rotating shift; overtime, unwanted, or "excessive" hours; two jobs; piecework versus hourly pay (pay mechanism influencing pace); fast pace of work, particularly in the presence of high vigilance demands; not enough time to complete work, deadlines; scheduling of work and rest cycles; variation in work load; and interruptions.
4. *Work content* (other than temporal aspects): Fractionated, repetitive, monotonous work, low task/skill variety; autonomy, independence, influence, control; utilization of existing skills; opportunity to learn new skills; mental alertness and concentration; unclear tasks or demands; conflicting tasks or demands; and insufficient resources, given work demands or responsibilities (e.g., skills, machinery, organizational structure).
5. *Interpersonal–work group:* Opportunity to interact with co-workers (during work, during breaks, after work); size, cohesiveness of primary work group; recognition for work performance; social support; instrumental support; and equitable work load.
6. *Interpersonal–supervision:* Participation in decision-making; receiving feedback and recognition from supervisor; providing supervisor with feed-

back; closeness of supervision; social support; instrumental support; and unclear, conflicting demands.

7. *Financial and economic aspects:* Pay, basic wages; additional compensation (overtime, shiftwork, bonuses); retirement benefits; other benefits (e.g., health care); and equity, predictability of compensation.
8. *Organizational aspects:* Size; structure (e.g., "flat" structure with relatively few levels in the organization); having a staff position (vs. line position); working on the boundary of the organization; relative prestige of the job; unclear organizational structure (lines of responsibility, organizational basis for role conflict and ambiguity); organizational (administrative) red tape and cumbersome (irrational) procedures; and discriminatory policies (e.g., hiring, promotion).
9. *Community and societal aspects:* This is not a category that is frequently considered, and thus it is much less clear what might turn out to be important. At minimum, we need to consider occupational status/prestige, since there are many studies showing an association (however opaque!) between status and health outcomes. Other considerations: Community perceptions of certain jobs (e.g., policemen) and their visibility (e.g., uniforms); community–company relations.
10. *Changes (or threatened changes) in the work setting:* Many of the dimensions listed above can undergo change, and such changes may also be worthy of our attention because of their possible impact on health. The kinds of changes that are likely to be important are often more global than dimensional: Promotion, demotion, loss of job, full-time to part-time transition, increased job insecurity, various organizational changes, and so on. The following cautions should be noted with respect to the study of change in the work setting: (a) In spite of the widespread presumption in the stress field that change per se is stressful, the evidence favors the stance that we should emphasize "negative" changes only (i.e., an aggravation along an already adverse or pathogenic work dimension, or global changes perceived as unwanted and undesirable). (b) Many changes in the work setting represent self-selection and are desired or sought; this makes it more difficult to determine the independent effects of such a change. (c) When change takes place from a less pathogenic environment to a more pathogenic one, then adverse impact of change per se is difficult to disentangle from the chronic effect of exposure to the latter environment. (d) We need to also pay attention to "non-changes" (above all, a promotion or desired transfer which fails to take place), since these may represent important stressors; detecting such "non-changes" is, of course, difficult.

In addition to the above listing of the dimensions of the work setting, it is important to consider, however tentatively, the *work–nonwork interface.* This has usually meant a consideration of the family roles of spouse and parent (e.g.,

Gutek et al., 1988; Repetti, 1987) and of the family setting with its own stress process and dynamics (e.g., Pearlin & Turner, 1987), but some investigators have also examined such issues as the impact of difficult rush hour commuting to and from work (Lundberg, 1976; Stokols & Novaco, 1981), recency of a vacation (Johansson, 1976), and the impact of work on political behavior and participation (Gardell, 1987; Levi, Frankenhaeuser, & Gardell, 1982) and leisure activities (Frankenhaeuser, 1977). However, the primary reason for bringing in the nonwork roles is that, from the perspective of impact of work on health, we wish to understand the underlying etiological dynamics whereby the daily impact of the pathogenic work situation becomes cumulative and health-threatening, rather than being daily defused and erased, thereby diminishing the expectation of a long-term adverse effect (Kasl, 1981). The lay concepts of "spillover" effects and unwinding, such as recovering from high arousal levels among female workers with unwanted overtime (Frankenhaeuser, 1979; Rissler, 1977), or among sawmill workers whose work is highly repetitious, machine paced, and highly constricting (Gardell, 1976; Johansson, Aronsson, & Lindstrom, 1978), are appropriate here. The nonwork roles, activities, and settings may act as buffers, or they may themselves represent an extension of the adverse impact of work. The issue thus far has been approached primarily from the social support perspective (e.g., Cohen & Syme, 1985) and we need to bring in many other structural and social-behavioral features of the family and social–leisure–recreational activities in order to expand our understanding of this area. For example, a cross-sectional survey of top-level male administrators (Burke, Weir, & DuWors, 1979) suggested complex dynamics involving the man's Type A behavior and high job commitment, the wife's higher depression and isolation, and her lower ability (readiness) to provide social support. And Vanfossen's (1981) data suggest the importance to the working husband of the work status of his wife: Working wives find intimacy in marriage (presumably a basis for mutual social support) less important and inequity (nonreciprocity in the relationship) more important.

Thus far I have listed work dimensions that are likely to impact on health. Documentation could be readily provided (see suggested earlier references) that associations have been reported between these dimensions and one or more of the following classes of outcomes: job satisfaction; absenteeism; indicators of distress, dysphoria, and psychophysiological symptoms; adverse lifestyle habits; biological indicators of arousal, distress, or risk of disease; illness behavior, seeking help or medical care; and health status indicators. The actual evidence, however, *must be delimited* in the following way. The indicators are not well interrelated and are, sometimes, uncorrelated. It is rare that a particular work dimension is found to associate with more than two or three of the above classes of indicators. And, of course, clearcut causal dynamics are rarely inferable. Above all, it must be emphasized that the evidence is not interchangeable: An impact in one area is not promissory of impact in another area, in most instances.

It is instructive to give a few illustrations of the last point above, since so many of us have been victimized by various stress formulations which confidently expect interchangeability of outcomes:

1. Cross-sectional analyses across a variety of occupations (Caplan et al., 1975; French et al., 1982) revealed a richness of significant associations among a number of work dimensions and a number of psychological strains, but biological variables such as blood pressure or cholesterol yielded overwhelmingly nonsignificant associations with either class of variables.
2. A recent study of bus drivers (Winkleby, Ragland, & Syme, 1988) revealed divergent associations with a carefully developed index of (self-reported) stressors: Negative association with hypertension but positive associations with gastrointestinal and respiratory problems.
3. Boring and monotonous work tasks do not seem to be associated with physiological arousal (Thackray, 1981), but adverse effects on job satisfaction and self-esteem are likely (Kasl, 1978).
4. Quantitative overload may be related to cardiovascular risk, while qualitative overload appears to have mental health consequences (Kasl, 1978, 1986).
5. Job loss and unemployment appear to have a definite long-term impact on depression (e.g., Dooley & Catalano, 1988), but the impact on cardiovascular functioning seems to be acute and self-limiting at best (Kasl & Cobb, 1980).

The evidence implicating specific health/disease outcomes in relation to specific work dimensions is neither plentiful nor systematic. For example, cause-specific mortality rates by occupational groups are not very informative, in several ways: (a) The independent variable does not pin down the specific work dimension involved; (b) we have little handle on self-selection factors, selective attrition factors, and on potential confounders (e.g., those related to broad social class issues); (c) the outcome variable, mortality, fails to narrow down the most probable pathway of influence, e.g., on risk factors versus on incidence of disease (independent of risk factors) versus on case fatality (independent of incidence).

Cardiovascular risk factors and cardiovascular disease hold center stage in research on occupational stress and specific work demands (e.g., Carruthers, 1980; Fletcher, 1988; House & Cottington, 1986). In contrast, occupational research on cancer is almost exclusively devoted to environmental exposures to carcinogens or ionizing radiation (e.g., Demopoulos & Mehlman, 1980; Schottenfeld & Fraumeni, 1982); this may be quite appropriate. Other specific conditions such as rheumatoid arthritis and peptic ulcer (Weiner, 1977), often viewed from a psychobiological perspective, are mostly approached in relation to personality traits and psychodynamic processes but not occupational variables. We have some occupational data on ulcers that suggest an excess among foremen (Pflanz, 1971; Susser, 1967), but the appropriate explanations for this are not obvious. Shiftworkers, especially on rotating shifts, tend to have an excess of gastrointestinal complaints (Rentos & Shepard, 1976; Tasto et al., 1978).

Occupational differences in coronary heart disease (CHD) mortality or mobidity (without a prospective design and without adjustments for potential confounders) are worth our attention when highly similar situations are being compared. This reduces the worry about confounders and narrows down the search for the specific pathogenic work dimension. For example (a) Benedictine priests working outside the monastery had a 65% higher rate of MI than Benedictine priests inside the monastery (Quinlan & Barrow, 1966); dietary factors were not an issue. (b) General practitioners had higher rates of MI than other physician groups (Morris, Heady, & Barley, 1952); differences in rates of cigarette smoking are a likely confounder in those old data on physicians (e.g., Russek, 1966). (c) In a study of NASA personnel (French & Caplan, 1970), CHD prevalence rates of managers were higher than those of scientists and engineers.

The formulation with respect to work and CHD that has received the most attention is that jobs and organizational roles that are associated with overload, excessive demands, and many responsibilities represent a setting of high CHD risk. The evidence (for review, see Kasl, 1986, and detailed citations therein) is a bit difficult to characterize. Certainly the formulation is viable and supportable, but detailed examination of evidence reveals various limitations. For example (a) Indicators such as holding two jobs, working overtime, or extra hours worked at home do not yield a consistent picture across studies. (b) Among male members of the Framingham cohort, only one work-related measure (number of promotions in the past 10 years) came in as a significant predictor in the multiple logistic regression (Haynes, Feinleib, & Kannel, 1980) but work overload did not. (c) It is not clear, particularly from the Swedish data (e.g., Alfredsson, Karasek, & Theorell, 1982), to what extent the overload or excessive demands are primarily psychological/mental, and how much physical demands play a role as well.

About 10 years ago, Karasek (1979) offered a formulation that had some promise of clarifying the above picture. In effect, he postulated that the dimension of work demands has to be considered jointly with *job decision latitude.* This leads us to a highly similar concept, *control*, which is attracting considerable attention both in the occupational area (e.g., Sauter et al., 1989) and in health psychology (e.g., Rodin, 1986). The concept of control in the work setting allows for a particularly instructive and pinpointed exploration of the issues involved in detecting and assessing exposure factors which impact on health. I draw on my recent review (Kasl, 1989) for the following comments on this area.

One of the first issues one runs into concerns the need to distinguish between control as an environmental characteristic and control as an evaluation or reaction (perceived control, sense of control). With respect to the former, definitions and appropriate measurements do not come easily. One can think of control as a response availability (linked to some aspect of work environment) to influence, in an intended direction, an important outcome. The potential overlap with other concepts is very high. For example, meeting job demands is certainly an important outcome; thus control facilitates meeting job demands, but since stress is most often defined as excess of demands over ability to meet them, *high control* begins to look suspiciously like *low stress.* Similarly, the concept of *resources in the environment* to meet job demands makes control overlap with *access to resources.* At the level of concrete work conditions, it is difficult to spell out what specific condition represents low control and how this differs from related dimensions such as monotony, repetitiveness, fractionation, pacing, close monitoring, and so on. In addition, as Smith (1985) has pointed out, these dimensions tend to be tightly interwoven and seldom can be studied in isolation.

With respect to the concept of control as an evaluation or reaction, rather than as an environmental condition, one quickly learns that (a) sense of control (locus of control, sense of efficacy) has trait-like characteristics, and workers' judgments of their work situation are likely to be influenced by this characteristic, which they bring to the job, and that (b) perceived control is richly linked to other variables, such as depression, low self-esteem, distress, poor adjustment, perceived stress, and so on, and cross-sectional associations among these variables no longer make a contribution to our knowledge. The primary contribution of the subjective or psychological version of the concept, control, should be to help us to answer the question, What are the health consequences of specific objective work conditions and are they modified or moderated by the subjective perceptions of control? I do not believe that so far we have any studies with the proper designs to tackle this question.

A close reading of the Swedish case-control and hospitalization studies (e.g., Alfredsson, 1985; Alfredsson, Karasek, & Theorell, 1982; Alfredsson, Spetz, & Theorell, 1985; Theorell, 1986) reveals a high CHD risk for jobs that are described both as "hectic" and as "few opportunities to learn." It is not clear that these are jobs with low discretion or control and that control is the crucial dimension. From an intervention perspective, we would like to know if we want to increase control over a boring, monotonous, repetitive job (and should it be through job redesign or is altering perception of control enough?), or do we want to effect a job enlargement (enrichment), because what is crucial is not the lack of control but the monotony?

There are other existing concepts in the organizational and occupational psychology literature that have their own accumulated empirical evidence, such as participation and autonomy (e.g., Breaugh, 1985; Gardell, 1982b; Spector, 1986). Just how the concept of control adds to these formulations and to this empirical evidence is not clear. Similarly, there is a reasonable, well-characterized empirical and conceptual literature on machine-paced and repetitive work (e.g., Cox, 1980, 1985; Smith, 1985). Is it appropriate to apply the concept of control, a higher order construct, to this body of evidence? What is it we don't understand about the processes described so that the concept of control will help us reinterpret or interpret better—will help us turn attention to other work situations that are generic to the concept of control but are not picked up by the notions of "repetitive" or "machine-paced"?

The concept of control, at least as applied to the work setting and its impact on health, cries out for the question "control over what?" But this question leads us back to the general issue: What aspects or dimensions impact on health? It is control in relation to those dimensions that is of interest to us. In other words, the concept of control and our measures of it need to be domain-specific. The following can be offered as some of the important ones: Scheduling of work (pace, deadlines, hours of work, periods of rest, etc.); influencing conditions at work; choosing methods for carrying out tasks; selecting resources that facilitate task completion; influencing performance evaluation, advancement, and job security; influencing interpersonal aspects of work, such as time and place to socialize with co-workers during work day; and choosing the content of one's work.

In effect, it appears that the most useful formulation may be to approach control as a subordinate construct, derivative of other dimensions. That is, we first identify the specific pathogenic conditions at work, and then we identify the mechanisms (e.g., design of machinery, company policy, nature of supervision, and so on) which alter or buffer the pathogenic conditions. Our concept of control is coordinated to the description of these mechanisms and is domain-specific. Instead, the literature offers us "control" as an overarching, superordinate construct, not tied down as an environmental condition nor as a cognitive or behavioral reaction, and inviting us to relabel old concepts and old findings in a more fashionable way.

AN OVERVIEW OF METHODOLOGICAL ISSUES IN DETECTING AND ASSESSING WORK-SETTING RISK FACTORS

In this concluding section, I wish to highlight what I consider to be the major methodological issues of research design strategy in studying the impact of work on health. A considerably more detailed discussion of these points has been given elsewhere (Kasl, 1985, 1986).

Fundamentally, we have a surfeit of studies that possess the following characteristics: (a) A cross-sectional design using self-report, paper-and-pencil measures; (b) a problematic separation between independent and dependent variables, due not only to the cross-sectional nature of the study but also because of measurement issues (e.g., conceptual and methodological overlap) and because of theoretical positions adopted (e.g., emphasis on intraperson cognitive processing); (c) an unmeasured and uncontrolled influence of preexisting stable characteristics of the person (e.g., neuroticism, negative affectivity, personal sense of efficacy, health problems); and (d) an undetermined anchoring to environmental exposures, on the one hand, and to physical health outcomes indexed by biomedical variables, on the other. There is no doubt that such studies rank high on convenience and feasibility. However, their contribution to already accumulated evidence may be minimal.

A number of areas suggest themselves as representing a likely contribution to the literature; I have chosen two of them for discussion in order to make illustrative points. Without doubt, these areas represent difficult challenges.

A Better Assessment of the Dimensions of Work Environment

Consider for a moment the measure of role ambiguity (Caplan et al., 1975), a major concept in occupational stress research. It contains four items dealing with clarity of job responsibilities and of work objectives, and with clarity and predictability of the expectations others have about the worker (respondent). The curious fact is that administrators—a group for whom the concept was practically invented—are quite a bit lower ($M = 2.06$, $SD = 0.88$) than such uncomplicated blue-collar occupations as forklift driver ($M = 2.74$, $SD = 1.29$) and machine tender ($M = 2.83$, $SD = 1.17$). Perhaps there are several culprits involved. Developing scales usable for all occupations makes the items rather vague and general. The anchoring in specific and concrete work conditions becomes intentionally obscure, and the items drift toward dealing with the respondents' cognitive processing and with reactions rather than simple description of environmental conditions. The respondents end up anchoring the items to various expectations and "levels of adaptation," which are based perhaps on personal experience and their judgments of how their jobs ought to be. Since respondents cannot be asked to judge their jobs in relation to other jobs (very few are that well informed), they should be asked to provide descriptive information in specific concrete terms.

As another example, consider the item, "Is your job hectic?" When asked of blue-collar workers in various assembly-line and machine-paced jobs it could reflect a specific aspect of pacing, plus some elements of quality control, and allowances for taking breaks. However, when the occupations also include managers, teachers, farmers, doctors, etc., then high-low scores on the total study population are very difficult to interpret. In fact, it is not implausible to suggest that those scoring high, but coming from a wide spectrum of jobs, are more likely to share common personal characteristics than common work-setting characteristics.

A Greater Commitment to the Importance of Biological Processes

I believe that there is an excessive emphasis on psychological formulations and on collection of psychological data, and an insufficient appreciation of the importance of biological processes and variables. Let me give a couple of examples. The first concerns the evidence from the broad literature on jobs involving quality control inspection (e.g., Drury, 1985) and clerical jobs involving computer application (e.g., Briner & Hockey, 1988; Turner & Karasek, 1984). Many of the jobs within this domain involve tight pacing, monotony, physical constraints, and need to maintain vigilance. Several studies (Haynes et al., 1985; Johansson & Aronsson, 1984; Wilkes, Stammerjohn, & Lalich, 1981) have reported rather similar findings: occupants of such jobs were higher on indices of strain/distress, but only if they performed such duties full-time. Elevated levels of strain were not observed among those performing those duties only part-time. It is possible that the best interpretation of these findings should be along the lines of physiological arousal, fatigue, and recovery, and cycles of work and rest. Workers may label the shorter task cycles as representing less control, but this may be only a phenomenological reconstruction, a mere epiphenomenon; it is the biological process of fatigue and recovery to which we may need to pay more attention.

The second example involves the literature on shiftwork (Rentos & Shepard, 1976; Tasto et al., 1978). If one zeros in specifically on the physiological data (Winget, Hughes, & LaDou, 1978), one becomes intrigued by the apparent importance of biomedical variables. For example, specific complaints, such as those regarding sleep, depend partly on individual differences in diurnal variations in levels of activity, such as preferring high levels of activity in the morning versus in the evening (Torsvall & Akerstedt, 1980). Psychosomatic complaints associated with night-work appear to be related to changes in serum gastrin levels, as well as to a stable trait variable, neuroticism (Akerstedt & Theorell, 1976).

A greater commitment to the value of biological indicators may sometimes lead to considerable difficulty regarding choice of variables. Fundamentally, we tend to work with either (a) indicators of arousal and reactivity, such as corticosteroids and catecholamines, or (b) known risk factors for specific diseases, such as blood pressure and serum cholesterol. The first set is more easily linked to environmental exposure than to disease outcomes, while the situation for the second set is reversed.

In the long run, it is likely we will need a somewhat different research paradigm for guiding our psychosocial studies in occupational epidemiology. At its best, the current paradigm (a) adopts a multiple risk factor approach to a particular disease, (b) accepts the need for prospective designs, (c) assesses work exposure variables together with biomedical risk factors, and (d) uses baseline data and multivariate analysis techniques to predict later development of disease among an initially healthy cohort.

In an enriched paradigm, we will need to develop research strategies so that the work exposure variable can be treated as a dynamic risk factor but can at the same time be entered into prospective analyses to predict disease outcomes. This implies the merging of short-term ipsative (within person) studies with long-term normative (across persons) disease outcome studies. An example will help here. In a study of blood pressure in the prison setting (Ostfeld, Kasl, D'Atri, & Fitzgerald, 1987) we found that blood pressure of prison guards increased significantly during a workday, and much more so in a maximum security prison than in a minimum one. Correctional treatment personnel also showed such a within-workday increase, particularly if they were female and had high contact with inmates. The point is that this shows variations in reactivity linked to variations in work setting, but we can't tell what the long-term risks are. Conversely, in the usual prospective epidemiological designs, these effects would not be detected. We need hybrid designs that will help us to understand how acute effects accumulate to produce long-term health threat—in what specific settings, on what vulnerable individuals, by what processes.

REFERENCES

Akerstedt, T., & Theorell, T. (1976). Exposure to night work: Serum gastrin reactions, psychosomatic complaints and personality variables. *Journal of Psychosomatic Research, 20,* 479–484.

Alfredsson, L. (1985). Myocardial infarction and environment. Use of registers in epidemiology. *Acta Medica Scandinavica,* Suppl. 698, 3–24.

Alfredsson, L., Karasek, R., & Theorell, T. (1982). Myocardial infarction risk and psychosocial work environment: An analysis of the male Swedish working force. *Social Science and Medicine, 16,* 463–467.

Alfredsson, L., Spetz, C.-L., & Theorell, T. (1985). Type of occupation and near future hospitalization for myocardial infarction and some other diagnoses. *International Journal of Epidemiology, 14,* 378–388.

Baker, D. B. (1985). The study of stress at work. *Annual Review of Public Health, 6,* 367–381.

Beehr, T. A., & Bhagat, R. S. (Eds.). (1985). *Human stress and cognition in organizations: An integrated perspective.* New York: Wiley.

Beehr, T. A., & Newman, J. E. (1978). Job stress, employee health, and organizational effectiveness: A facet analysis, model, and literature review. *Personnel Psychology, 31,* 665–699.

Brady, J. V., & Fischman, M. W. (1986). Biobehavioral principles, behavioral medicine, and the workplace. In M. F. Cataldo & T. J. Coates (Eds.), *Health and industry: A behavioral medicine perspective* (pp. 9–17). New York: Wiley.

Breaugh, J. A. (1985). The measurement of work autonomy. *Human Relations, 38,* 551–570.

Briner, R., & Hockey, G. R. J. (1988). Operator stress and computer-based work. In C. L. Cooper & R. Payne (Eds.), *Causes, coping, and consequences of stress at work* (pp. 115–140). Chichester: Wiley.

Burke, R. J. (Ed.). (1984). *Current issues in occupational stress: Research and intervention.* Downsview, Ontario: Faculty of Administrative Studies, York University.

Burke, R. J., Weir, T., & DuWors, R. E., Jr. (1979). Type A behavior of administrators and wives' reports of marital satisfaction and well-being. *Journal of Applied Psychology, 64,* 57–65.

Caplan, R. D., Cobb, S., French, F. R. P., Jr., Harrison, R. V., & Pinneau, S. R., Jr. (1975). *Job demands and worker health* (HEW Publication No. [NIOSH] 75-160). Washington, DC: U.S. Government Printing Office.

Carruthers, M. (1980). Hazardous occupations and the heart. In C. L. Cooper & R. Payne (Eds.), *Current concerns in occupational stress* (pp. 3–22). Chichester: Wiley.

Cataldo, M. F., & Coates, T. J. (Eds.). (1986). *Health & industry: A behavioral medicine perspective.* New York: Wiley.

Cattell, R. B. (1957). *Personality and motivation structure and measurement.* Yonkers: World Book.

Chinoy, E. (1955). *Automobile workers and the American dream.* Garden City, NY: Doubleday.

Cohen, S., & Syme, S. L. (Eds.). (1985). *Social support and health.* Orlando: Academic Press.

Cooper, C. L., Davidson, M. J., & Robinson, P. (1982). Stress in the police service. *Journal of Occupational Medicine, 24,* 31–36.

Cooper, C. L., & Marshall, J. (Eds.). (1980). *White collar and professional stress.* Chichester: Wiley.

Cooper, C. L., & Payne, R. (Eds.). (1978). *Stress at work.* Chichester: Wiley.

Cooper, C. L., & Payne, R. (Eds.). (1980). *Current concerns in occupational stress.* Chichester: Wiley.

Cooper, C. L., & Payne, R. (Eds.). (1988). *Causes, coping and consequences of stress at work.* Chichester: Wiley.

Cooper, C. L., & Smith, M. J. (Eds.). (1985). *Job stress and blue collar work.* Chichester: Wiley.

Cox, T. (1980). Repetitive work. In C. L. Cooper & R. Payne (Eds.), *Current concerns in occupational stress* (pp. 23–41). Chichester: Wiley.

Cox, T. (1985). Repetitive work. Occupational stress and health. In C. L. Cooper & M. J. Smith (Eds.), *Job stress and blue collar work* (pp. 85–112). Chichester: Wiley.

Crump, J. H. (1979). Review of stress in air traffic control: Its measurement and effects. *Aviation, Space, and Environmental Medicine, 50,* 243–248.

Davidson, M. J., & Veno, A. (1980). Stress and the policeman. In C. L. Cooper & J. Marshall (Eds.), *White collar and professional stress* (pp. 131–166). Chichester: Wiley.

Demopoulos, H. B., & Mehlman, M. A. (Eds.). (1980). *Cancer and the environment.* Park Forest South, Illinois: Photox Publishers.

Dooley, D., & Catalano, R. (Eds.). (1988). Psychological effects of unemployment. *Journal of Social Issues, 44,* 1–191.

Drury, C. G. (1985). Stress and quality control inspection. In C. L. Cooper & M. J. Smith (Eds.), *Job stress and blue collar work* (pp. 113–129). Chichester: Wiley.

Dunnette, M. D. (Ed.). (1976). *Handbook of industrial and organizational psychology.* Chicago: Rand McNally.

Elliott, G. R., & Eisdorfer, C. (Eds.). (1982). *Stress and human health.* New York: Springer.

Evans, G. W. (Ed.). (1982). *Environmental stress.* New York: Cambridge University Press.

Fimian, M. J. (1984). The development of an instrument to measure occupational stress in teachers: The Teacher Stress Inventory. *Journal of Occupational Psychology, 57,* 277–293.

Fletcher, B. C. (1988). The epidemiology of occupational stress. In C. L. Cooper & R. Payne (Eds.), *Causes, coping and consequences of stress at work* (pp. 3–50). Chichester: Wiley.

Frankenhaeuser, M. (1977). Job demands, health, and well being. *Journal of Psychosomatic Research, 21,* 313–321.

Frankenhaeuser, M. (1979). Psychoneuroendocrine approaches to the study of emotion as related to stress and coping. In H. E. Howe & R. A. Dienstbier (Eds.), *Nebraska Symposium on Motivation* (pp. 123–161). Lincoln: University of Nebraska Press.

French, J. R. P., Jr., & Caplan, R. D. (1970). Psychosocial factors in coronary heart disease. *Industrial Medicine and Surgery, 39,* 383–397.

French, J. R. P., Jr., Caplan, R. D., & Van Harrison, R. (1982). *The mechanisms of job stress and strain.* Chichester: Wiley.

Frese, M., & Zapf, D. (1988). Methodological issues in the study of work stress: Objective vs. subjective measurement of work stress and the question of longitudinal studies. In C. L. Cooper & R. Payne (Eds.), *Causes, coping, and consequences of stress at work* (pp. 375–411). Chichester: Wiley.

Gardell, B. (1976). *Job content and quality of life.* Stockholm: Prisma.

Gardell, B. (1982a). Scandinavian research on stress in working life. *International Journal of Health Services, 12,* 31–41.

Gardell, B. (1982b). Worker participation and autonomy: A multilevel approach to democracy at the workplace. *International Journal of Health Services, 12,* 527–558.

Gardell, B. (1987). Efficiency and health hazards in mechanized work. In J. C. Quick, R. S. Bhagat, J. E. Dalton, & J. D. Quick (Eds.), *Work stress: Health care systems in the workplace* (pp. 50–71). New York: Praeger.

Geddes, R., & Gutman, R. (1977). The assessment of the built environment for safety: Research and practice. In L. E. Hinkle, Jr., & W. C. Loring (Eds.), *The effect of the man-made environment on health and behavior* (pp. 143–195). Centers for Disease Control, Atlanta: DHEW Publication No. (CDC) 77-8318.

Gentry, W. D., & Parkes, K. R. (1982). Psychological stress in intensive care unit and non-intensive care nursing: A review of the past decade. *Heart & Lung, 11,* 43–47.

Gray-Toft, P., & Anderson, J. G. (1981). The nursing stress scale: Development of an instrument. *Journal of Behavioral Assessment, 3,* 11–23.

Gutek, B. A., Repetti, R. L., & Silver, D. L. (1988). Nonwork roles and stress at work. In C. L. Cooper & R. Payne (Eds.), *Causes, coping and consequences of stress at work* (pp. 141–174). Chichester: Wiley.

Hackman, J. R., & Oldham, G. R. (1975). Development of the Job Diagnostic Survey. *Journal of Applied Psychology, 60,* 159–170.

Haynes, S. G., Feinleib, M., & Kannel, W. B. (1980). The relationship of psychosocial factors to coronary heart disease in the Framingham Study: III. Eight-year incidence of coronary heart disease. *American Journal of Epidemiology, 111,* 37–58.

Haynes, S. G., LaCroix, A. Z., & Lippin, T. (1987). The effect of high job demands and low control on the health of employed women. In J. C. Quick, R. S. Bhagat, J. E. Dalton, & J. D. Quick (Eds.), *Work stress: Health care systems in the work place* (pp. 93–110). New York: Praeger.

Hicks, W. D., & Klimoski, R. J. (1981). The impact of flextime on employee attitudes. *Academy of Management Journal, 24,* 333–341.

Holt, R. R. (1982). Occupational stress. In L. Goldberger & S. Breznitz (Eds.), *Handbook of stress* (pp. 419–444). New York: The Free Press.

House, J. S. (1980). *Occupational stress and mental and physical health of factory workers.* Ann Arbor: ISR Research Report.

House, J. S. (1981). *Work stress and social support.* Reading: Addison-Wesley.

House, J. S., & Cottington, E. M. (1986). Health and the workplace. In L. H. Aiken & D. Mechanic (Eds.), *Applications of Social Science to Clinical Medicine and Health Policy* (pp. 392–416). New Brunswick: Rutgers University Press.

Hurrell, J. J., and Colligan, M. J. (1982). Psychological job stress. In W. N.

Rom (Ed.), *Environmental and occupational medicine* (pp. 425–430). Boston: Little, Brown, & Co.

Jenkins, C. D., DeFrank, R. S., & Speers, M. A. (1984). *Evaluation of psychometric methodologies used to assess occupational stress and strain.* Galveston, Texas: Department of Preventive Medicine and Community Health, University of Texas Medical Branch.

Jenkins, G. D., Nadler, D. A., Lawler, E. E., III, & Cammann, C. (1975). Standardized observation: An approach to measuring the nature of jobs. *Journal of Applied Psychology, 60,* 171–181.

Jick, T. D., & Burke, R. J. (1982). Occupational stress: Recent findings and new directions. *Journal of Occupational Behaviour, 3,* 1–3.

Johansson, G. (1976). Subjective wellbeing and temporal patterns of sympathetic adrenal medullary activity. *Biological Psychology, 4,* 157–172.

Johansson, G., & Aronsson, G. (1984). Stress reactions in computerized administrative work. *Journal of Occupational Behaviour, 5,* 159–181.

Johansson, G., Aronsson, G., & Lindstrom, B. P. (1978). Social psychological and neuroendocrine stress reactions in highly mechanized work. *Ergonomics, 21,* 583–599.

Jones, D. M., & Chapman, A. J. (Eds.). (1984). *Noise and society.* Chichester: Wiley.

Kahn, R. L. (1981). *Work and Health.* New York: Wiley.

Kahn, R. L. (1987). Work stress in the 1980's: Research and practice. In J. C. Quick, R. S. Bhagat, J. E. Dalton, & J. D. Quick (Eds.), *Work stress: Health care systems in the workplace* (pp. 311–320). New York: Praeger.

Kahn, R. L., Hein, K., House, J., Kasl, S. V., & McLean, A. A. (1982). Report on stress in organizational settings. In G. R. Elliott & C. Eisdorfer (Eds.), *Stress and human health* (pp. 81–117). New York: Springer.

Kahn, R. L., Wolfe, D. M., Quinn, R. P., Snoek, J. D., & Rosenthal, R. A. (1964). *Organizational stress: Studies in role conflict and ambiguity.* New York: Wiley.

Karasek, R. A., Jr. (1979). Job demands, job decision latitude, and mental strain: Implications for job redesign. *Administrative Science Quarterly, 24,* 285–308.

Karasek, R. A., Theorell, T., Schwartz, J. E., Schnall, P. L., Pieper, C. F., & Michela, J. L. (1988). Job characteristics in relation to the prevalence of myocardial infarction in the US Health Examination Survey (HES) and the Health and Nutrition Examination Survey (HANES). *American Journal of Public Health, 78,* 910–918.

Kasl, S. V. (1974). Work and mental health. In J. O'Toole (Ed.), *Work and the quality of life* (pp. 171–196). Cambridge: The MIT Press.

Kasl, S. V. (1978). Epidemiological contributions to the study of work stress. In C. L. Cooper & R. Payne (Eds.), *Stress at work* (pp. 3–48). Chichester: Wiley.

Kasl, S. V. (1981). The challenge of studying the disease effects of stressful work conditions. *American Journal of Pubic Health, 71,* 682–684.

Kasl, S. V. (1983). Pursuing the link between stressful life experiences and disease: A time for re-appraisal. In C. L. Cooper (Ed.), *Stress research: Issues for the eighties* (pp. 79–102). Chichester: Wiley.

Kasl, S. V. (1984). Stress and health. *Annual Review of Public Health, 5,* 319–341.

Kasl, S. V. (1985). Environmental exposure and disease: An epidemiological perspective on some methodological issues in health psychology and behavioral medicine. In A. Baum & J. E. Singer (Eds.), *Advances in environmental psychology: Vol. 5. Methods and environmental psychology* (pp. 119–146). Hillsdale, NJ: Erlbaum.

Kasl, S. V. (1986). Stress and disease in the workplace: A methodological commentary on the accumulated evidence. In M. F. Cataldo & T. J. Coates (Eds.), *Health and industry: A behavioral medicine perspective* (pp. 52–85). New York: Wiley.

Kasl, S. V. (1989). An epidemiological perspective on the role of control in health. In S. L. Sauter, J. J. Hurrell, Jr., & C. L. Cooper (Eds.), *Job control and worker health* (pp. 161–189). Chichester: Wiley.

Kasl, S. V., Chisholm, R. F., & Eskenazi, B. (1981). The impact of the accident at the Three Mile Island on the behavior and well-being of nuclear workers. *American Journal of Public Health, 71,* 472–495.

Kasl, S. V., & Cobb, S. (1980). The experience of losing a job: Some effects on cardiovascular functioning. *Psychotherapy and Psychosomatics, 34,* 88–109.

Kasl, S. V., & Cobb, S. (1983). Psychological and social stresses in the workplace. In B. S. Levy & D. H. Wegman (Eds.), *Occupational health* (pp. 251–263). Boston: Little, Brown, & Co.

Kates, R. W., & Wohlwill, J. F. (Ed.). (1966). Man's response to the physical environment. *Journal of Social Issues, 22*(4), 1–136.

Kornhauser, A. (1965). *Mental health of the industrial worker.* New York: Wiley.

Krausz, M., & Freibach, N. (1983). Effects of flexible working time for employed women upon satisfaction, strains and absenteeism. *Journal of Occupational Psychology, 56,* 155–159.

Levi, L., Frankenhaeuser, M., & Gardell, B. (1982). Report on work stress related to social structures and processes. In G. R. Elliott & C. Eisdorfer (Eds.), *Stress and human health* (pp. 119–146). New York: Springer.

Levy, B. S., & Wegman, D. H. (Eds.). (1983). *Occupational health.* Boston: Little, Brown, & Co.

Locke, E. A. (1976). The nature and causes of job satisfaction. In M. D. Dunnette (Ed.), *Handbook of industrial and organizational psychology* (pp. 1297–1349). Chicago: Rand McNally.

Lundberg, U. (1976). Urban commuting: Crowdedness and catecholamine excretion. *Journal of Human Stress, 2*, 26–32.

Matteson, M. T., & Ivancevich, J. M. (1982). Stress and the medical technologist: I. A general overview. *American Journal of Medical Technology, 48*, 163–168.

McGrath, J. E. (1970). A conceptual formulation for research on stress. In J. E. McGrath (Ed.), *Social and psychological factors in stress* (pp. 10–21). New York: Holt, Rinehart, and Winston.

McGrath, J. E. (1976). Stress and behavior in organizations. In M. D. Dunnette (Ed.), *Handbook of industrial and organizational psychology* (pp. 1351–1395). Chicago: Rand McNally.

McLean, A. A. (1979). *Work stress.* Reading: Addison-Wesley.

Miles, R. H. (1980). Boundary roles. In C. L. Cooper & R. Payne (Eds.), *Current concerns in occupational stress* (pp. 61–96). Chichester: Wiley.

Morris, J. N., Heady, J. A., & Barley, R. G. (1952). Coronary heart disease in medical practitioners. *British Journal of Medicine, 1*, 503–520.

Narayanan, V. K., & Nath, R. (1982). A field test of some attitudinal and behavioral consequences of flextime. *Journal of Applied Psychology, 67*, 214–218.

Office of Technology Assessment. (1985). *Automation of America's offices 1985–2000.* Washington, DC: U.S. Government Printing Office.

Ostfeld, A. M., Kasl, S. V., D'Atri, D. A., & Fitzgerald, E. F. (1987). *Stress, crowding, and blood pressure in prison.* Hillsdale, NJ: Erlbaum.

Pearlin, L. I., & Turner, H. A. (1987). The family as a context of the stress process. In S. V. Kasl & C. L. Cooper (Eds.), *Stress and health: Issues in research methodology* (pp. 143–165). Chichester: Wiley.

Pelz, D., & Andrews, F. (1966). *Scientists in organizations.* New York: Wiley.

Pflanz, M. (1971). Epidemiological and sociocultural factors in the etiology of duodenal ulcer. In H. Weiner (Ed.), *Advances in psychosomatic medicine: Vol. 6. Duodenal Ulcer* (pp. 121–151). Basel: Karger.

Phillips, B. N., & Lee, M. (1980). The changing role of the American teacher: Current and future sources of stress. In C. L. Cooper & J. Marshall (Eds.), *White collar and professional stress* (pp. 93–111). Chichester: Wiley.

Pooling Project Research Group. (1978). Relationship of blood pressure, serum cholesterol, smoking habit, relative weight and ECG abnormalities to incidence of major coronary events. Final report of pooling project. *Journal of Chronic Diseases, 31*, 201–306.

Quick, J. C., Bhagat, R. S., Dalton, J. E., & Quick, J. D. (Eds.). (1987). *Work stress: Health care systems in the workplace.* New York: Praeger.

Quinlan, C. B., & Barrow, J. G. (1966). Prevalence of coronary heart disease in Trappist and Benedictine monks. *Circulation, 33–34* (Suppl. III), 193.

Quinn, R. P., & Shepard, L. J. (1974). *The 1972–73 quality of employment survey.* Ann Arbor: Institute for Social Research.

Quinn, R., Seashore, S., Kahn, R., Mangione, T., Campbell, D., Staines, G., & McCullough, M. (1971). *Survey of working conditions* (Document No. 2916-0001). Washington, DC: U.S. Government Printing Office.

Rentos, G. P., & Shepard, R. D. (Eds.). (1976). *Shift work and health, A symposium.* Washington, DC: DHEW (NIOSH) Publication No. 76-203.

Repetti, R. L. (1987). Linkages between work and family roles. In S. Oskamp (Ed.), *Applied Social Psychology Annual: Vol. 7. Family Processes and Problems* (pp. 98–127). Beverly Hills: Sage.

Rissler, A. (1977). Stress reactions at work and after work during a period of quantitative overload. *Ergonomics, 20,* 13–16.

Robinson, J. P., Athanasiou, R., & Head, K. B. (Eds.). (1969). *Measures of occupational attitudes and occupational characteristics.* Ann Arbor, Michigan: Institute for Social Research.

Rodin, J. (1986). Aging and health: Effects of the sense of control. *Science, 233,* 1271–1276.

Rose, R. M., Jenkins, C. D., & Hurst, M. W. (1978). *Air traffic controller health change study.* Boston University School of Medicine: A report to the FAA, Contract No. DOT-FA72WA-3211.

Russek, H. J. (1966). Stress, tobacco, and coronary disease in North American professional groups. *Journal of the American Medical Association, 192,* 189–194.

Salvendy, G., & Smith, M. J. (Eds.). (1981). *Machine pacing and occupational stress.* London: Taylor & Francis.

Sauter, S. L., Hurrell, J. J., Jr., & Cooper, C. L. (Eds.). (1989). *Job control and worker health.* Chichester: Wiley.

Schottenfeld, D., & Fraumeni, J. F., Jr. (Eds.). (1982). *Cancer epidemiology and prevention.* Philadelphia: W. B. Saunders.

Sethi, A. S., & Schuler, R. S. (Eds.). (1984). *Handbook of organizational stress coping strategies.* Cambridge, MA: Ballinger.

Sharit, J., & Salvendy, G. (1982). Occupational stress: Review and appraisal. *Human Factors, 24,* 129–162.

Shephard, R. J. (1974). *Men at work.* Springfield, IL: C. C. Thomas.

Shostak, A. B. (1980). *Blue-collar stress.* Reading: Addison-Wesley.

Smith, F. J. (1976). Index of organizational reactions (IOR). *JSAS Catalog of Selected Documents in Psychology, 6:* 54, No. 1265.

Smith, M. J. (1985). Machine-paced work and stress. In C. L. Cooper & M. J. Smith (Eds.), *Job stress and blue collar work* (pp. 51–64). Chichester: Wiley.

Smith, P. C., Kendall, L. M., & Hulin, C. L. (1969). *The measurement of satisfaction in work and retirement.* Chicago: Rand McNally.

Spector, P. E. (1986). Perceived control by employees: A meta-analysis of studies concerning autonomy and participation at work. *Human Relations, 39,* 1005–1016.

Stellman, J. M., & Snow, B. R. (1986). Occupational safety and health hazards and the psychosocial health and well-being of workers. In M. F. Cataldo & T. J. Coates (Eds.), *Health and industry: A behavioral medicine perspective.* (pp. 270–284). New York: Wiley.

Steptoe, A., & Mathews, A. (Eds.). (1984). *Health care and human behaviour.* London: Academic Press.

Stokols, D., and Novaco, R. W. (1981). Transportation and well-being: An ecological perspective. In I. Altman, J. Wohlwill, & P. Everett (Eds.), *Transportation environments.* New York: Plenum Press.

Susser, M. (1967). Causes of peptic ulcer: A selective epidemiologic review. *Journal of Chronic Diseases, 20,* 435–456.

Tasto, D., Colligan, M. J., Skjei, E. W., & Polly, S. J. (1978). *Health consequences of shiftwork.* DHEW (NIOSH) Publication No. 78-154. Washington, DC: U.S. Government Printing Office.

Thackray, R. I. (1981). The stress of boredom and monotony: A consideration of the evidence. *Psychosomatic Medicine, 43,* 165–176.

Theorell, T. (1986). Stress at work and risk of myocardial infarction. *Postgraduate Medical Journal, 62,* 791–795.

Torsvall, L., & Akerstedt, T. (1980). A diurnal type scale: Construction, consistency and validation in shift work. *Scandinavian Journal of Work Environment and Health, 6,* 283–290.

Turner, J. A., & Karasek, R. A. (1984). Software ergonomics: Effects of computer application design parameters on operator task performance and health. *Ergonomics, 27,* 663–690.

U.S. Department of Commerce. (1980). *Standard occupational classification manual.* Washington, DC: Superintendent of Documents, U.S. Government Printing Office.

Vanfossen, B. E. (1981). Sex differences in the mental health effects of spouse support and equity. *Journal of Health and Social Behavior, 22,* 130–143.

Weiner, H. (1977). *Psychobiology and human disease.* New York: Elsevier.

Weiss, D. S., Davis, R. V., England, G. W., & Lofquist, L. H. (1967). *Manual for the Minnesota Satisfaction Questionnaire.* Minneapolis: University of Minnesota Industrial Relations Center.

Wilkes, B., Stammerjohn, L., & Lalich, N. (1981). Job demands and worker health in machine-paced poultry inspection. *Scandinavian Journal of Work Environment and Health, 7* (Suppl. 4), 12–19.

Winget, C. M., Hughes, L., & LaDou, J. (1978). Physiological effects of rotational work shifting: A review. *Journal of Occupational Medicine, 20,* 204–210.

Winkleby, M. A., Ragland, D. R., & Syme, S. L. (1988). Self-reported stressors and hypertension: Evidence of an inverse association. *American Journal of Epidemiology, 127,* 124–134.

5

THE ROLE OF THE PHYSICAL ENVIRONMENT IN THE HEALTH AND WELL-BEING OF CHILDREN

Gary W. Evans
Wendy Kliewer
Janaea Martin

University of California, Irvine

INTRODUCTION

This chapter describes how the physical environment can influence the behavior of children. We focus on underlying dimensions of physical settings that operate across a range of environmental conditions, including crowding, pollutants, noise, and architectural design. Six underlying dimensions of the physical environment are examined. These dimensions include pathogenic conditions, stimulation levels, functional complexity, control, structure and predictability, and exploration.

Pathogenic conditions directly affect organism structure and functioning. Typically, human research on pathogenic environmental conditions has emphasized toxic effects or nonspecific, psychophysiological stress responses. Stimulation levels refer to the amount of physical information impinging upon the organism. As we suggest, either too little or too much background physical stimulation may be harmful to developing children. Functional complexity describes the characteristics of more proximate, focal objects such as toys or learning materials. Functional complexity has been operationalized primarily in terms of object variety or responsiveness. Environments vary in the degree of

This chapter was written while the senior author was Visiting Professor in the Psychology Division, Department of Psychiatry, Karolinska Institute, Stockholm, Sweden. We thank Ulf Lundberg and Marianne Frankenhaeuser for generous institutional support. Preparation of this chapter was also supported by Training Grant T32 MH 16868 from the National Institute of Mental Health. We thank Harry Heft and Carol Weinstein for critical feedback on earlier drafts of this chapter.

control they afford children. Prolonged exposure to uncontrollable conditions in the home or school setting may affect the development of self-efficacy in younger children. Predictability and structure reflect the degree of underlying order and coherence in the physical environment. Finally, exploration refers to the degree to which the child is able to actively move around in his or her environment.

Our analysis is limited to children because of page restrictions and because we believe the health and well-being of children, in comparison with adults, are often more severely affected by the quality of the physical environment. Our analysis of children and the physical environment includes the period from conception to late elementary school. The chapter emphasizes assessment and is not an exhaustive treatment of the literature on children and the physical environment. For more complete reviews see Parke (1978), Wachs and Gruen (1982), Weinstein and David (1987), and Wohlwill and Heft (1987). After the dimensions of the physical environment and their assessment are explained, their interrelations are described. This is followed by a more general discussion of conceptual issues. The final section of the chapter addresses how the physical environment can promote better health in children.

DIMENSIONS OF THE PHYSICAL ENVIRONMENT

Pathogenic Conditions

Pollutants

Recently, scientific attention has increased in three areas of research on children and pollutants: (a) Passive exposure to cigarette smoke, (b) the sick building syndrome, and (c) behavioral teratology. Passive exposure to cigarette smoke in the home increases risk for lung cancer in children. These children also have higher rates of respiratory disorders and middle ear effusions (National Academy of Sciences, 1986).

Children are also susceptible to the sick building syndrome. For example, higher than expected medical complaints have been noted in staff and children in about 20% of preschools built in the Stockholm area since 1975. These complaints include sensory irritation, skin rashes, mental fatigue, and weak but persistent odors (Berglund & Lindvall, 1986). Attempts to uncover the physical basis for such buildings have been largely unsuccessful, although it is clear the syndrome is a by-product of the tightening of buildings for energy conservation purposes. Very little is known about children's reactions to other indoor pollutants emanating from cooking and heating fixtures (e.g., gas stoves) or from building materials (e.g., formaldehyde).

Psychologists are also becoming interested in *behavioral teratology,* the study of early toxic exposures on development. Most of this work has focused on the study of heavy metals such as lead and mercury as they affect human health and behavior. It is largely because of behavioral research on the effects of chronic exposure to low levels of ambient lead on developing children that current legislation in many parts of the world has dramatically lowered permissible ambient lead levels.

Acute lead poisoning causes neuropathology associated with encephalopathy, severe gastritis and colic, weakness in the joints, and high levels of mortality in children (Rutter, 1980; Weiss, 1983). Interest in the behavioral effects of lead was first aroused by data indicating that young children hospitalized for lead poisoning and then released with no clinical symptoms, 2 to 8 years later suffered IQ deficits, behavioral problems, and difficulties in school (Byers & Lord, 1943). Although this study had no control groups and is subject to some alternative interpretations (e.g., most of the children were from economically deprived backgrounds), subsequent research found similar, delayed behavioral and cognitive deficits in children initially the victims of lead poisoning (Rutter, 1980).

An important remaining question is whether chronic lead exposure, not overtly toxic, can also be harmful to children. Here too there is growing evidence of teratological effects. Needleman and his associates analyzed dental lead levels from a large urban sample of children who had no clinical symptoms of lead toxicity. Comparing the upper and lower deciles of lead dentition concentrations, they found significant reductions in IQ and psychomotor performance, and higher ratings of behavioral disturbance in the classroom of those students in the upper decile (Needleman et al., 1979). Similar behavioral deficits have been found in other urban populations of children with above normal body burdens of lead (Rutter, 1980). Moreover, parallel findings have been noted in primate studies with controlled exposure to lead through diet (Weiss, 1983).

Minimata disease or acute methylmercury poisoning is named after a Japanese fishing village that was the scene of epidemic mercury poisoning caused by industrial dumping in Minimata Bay. Many adults and children ingesting fish at the time of the industrial dumping suffered signs of acute mercury toxicity including severe tremors, central nervous system impairment, and in some cases death. Children who were exposed to toxins in utero had significantly lower IQs, and retarded speech and motor development (Fein, Schwartz, Jacobson, & Jacobson, 1983). Tragically, other outbreaks of Minimata disease following ingestion of mercury-contaminated foodstuffs have been documented in other countries (Weiss, 1983). It is noteworthy that 22 out of the 23 documented cases of in utero exposure at Minimata showed no overt signs of clinical toxicity in the mothers. Delayed effects of toxin exposure were manifested in children even when no clinical symptoms of damage were present in their mothers during the gestation period.

Perhaps more significant is evidence that exposure of mothers to some toxins prior to conception can have latent, behavioral effects on their children. For example, mothers who ingest polychlorinated biphenyls (PCBs) prior to conception are more likely to bear children with retarded intellectual and psychomotor development (Fein et al., 1983). One of the problems with PCBs is that they are fat soluble and easily stored in mammalian tissue. For example, PCB levels in the spinal cord and breast milk are correlated with rates of fish ingestion from women living near Lake Michigan. These PCB measurements, in turn, are related to deficits in visual recognition memory, motor immaturity, and slower reflex responses in young children of these mothers (Jacobson, Jacobson, Fein, Schwartz, & Dowler, 1984).

Noise

There is limited evidence for direct pathogenic effects in children exposed to chronic noise. Children in schools near noise sources have elevated blood pressure. Karsdorf and Klappach (1968) found increased systolic and diastolic blood pressure in seventh through tenth graders in two schools proximate to noisy urban streets. Likewise Karagodina, Soldatkina, Vinokur, and Klimukhin (1969) found abnormally high blood pressure in children residing around nine different Soviet airports. Unfortunately, neither of these studies provides sufficient information on subject characteristics to judge how well matched the samples were. More recently, Cohen and his colleagues compared the responses of children attending noisy schools in the Los Angeles airport area to children from similar but relatively quiet school areas. In addition to matching children on socioeconomic background, these researchers also statistically controlled for parental occupation, parental education, and, height and weight of each child. Their analyses indicate small but significant increases in blood pressure associated with noise exposure at school. Furthermore, these noise-related elevations in blood pressure do not habituate with continued noise exposure across a 5-year span (Cohen, Evans, Krantz, & Stokols, 1980; Cohen, Evans, Krantz, Stokols, & Kelly, 1982; Cohen, Evans, Stokols, & Krantz, 1986).

Crowding

There are more limited data suggesting a possible link between high density levels with poorer health in children. Children of ages 9 through 17 years evidenced increased skin conductance in a short-term laboratory experiment on crowding (Aiello, Nicosia, & Thompson, 1979). Boys in particular reacted strongly. Children from higher density homes have higher rates of illness (Booth & Johnson, 1975), but methodological problems and conflicting data from other studies (Baum & Paulus, 1987; Evans, 1978) make it impossible to draw any firm conclusions about the association between residential density and children's physical health.

Summary

Pollutants, noise, and crowding may affect children's physical health. In addition to overt pathological symptoms, toxins may have subtle, long-lasting effects on the neural systems of developing organisms. Chronic exposure to noise and possibly to crowding can affect cardiovascular functioning in children.

Assessment of outcome measures from exposure to pathogenic environmental conditions raises several interesting issues. Some reactions may be specific to a particular environmental condition, while others may be more general. For example, noise causes deficits in auditory functioning, whereas crowding has no known auditory effects. Yet both of these environmental conditions can elevate blood pressure and, at least in adults, also raise neuroendocrine (e.g., adrenaline) levels during acute exposures (Evans & Cohen, 1987). Moreover, many behavioral toxins produce general malaise consisting of allergic reactions, fatigue, and lethargy. On the other hand, unique effects also occur that are toxin-specific. These various patterns of specific and nonspecific physiological responses to pathogenic environmental conditions imply that multimethod assessment strategies are necessary to accurately measure the range and quality of environmental effects on children.

Another difficult assessment problem is the estimation of exposure to environmental pathogens (Evans & Tafalla, 1987). Children move through many settings in the course of a day. They spend time outdoors as well as indoors and perhaps travel in a car or bus. Even when exposure can be reasonably well estimated, it is not clear what metric should be used. For example, in measuring noise, should exposure to peak levels be monitored, average energy functions over the day, or weighted averages that include night exposure adjustments? In the case of crowding, we know that estimates of indoor crowding (e.g., people per room) are associated with different outcome variables than are external crowding measures (e.g., people per acre) (van Vliet, 1985). Furthermore, should estimates of current exposure be utilized or an assessment of chronic effects? Finally, as noted earlier, some pathogens have immediate effects on health, whereas others have more delayed effects. Concurrent measurement of environmental effects on children's health and well-being may overlook important, cumulative impacts that take time to manifest themselves. Both synchronous and lagged relations between environmental conditions and outcome measures are often called for.

Stimulation

The amount of physical stimulation impinging upon the organism has long interested psychologists. Hebb's (1949) neural net theory suggested that cortical development was influenced by physical stimulation during maturation. This theory led to a large literature on the effects of early experience on the developing neural system of animals. Most of this work examined what happens when either too little stimulation is available or when certain aspects of stimulation are systematically distorted (Thompson & Grusec, 1970). One of the implications of Hebb's theory is, the more stimulation the better. Thus stimulation could be thought of on a linear continuum ranging from deprivation to enrichment. More recent conceptualizations of stimulation view the relationship of stimulation levels and well-being as an inverted-U shape function with moderate levels as optimal (Wohlwill, 1974).

Some of the negative effects of noise and crowding on human development may be due to stimulus overload. Heightened sound levels and the close presence of people may increase the amount of visual, auditor, thermal, and olfactory stimulation impinging upon the organism.

Noise

In a program of research investigating influences of the home social and physical environment on early child development, Wachs and colleagues have accumulated data across several studies showing a negative association between home noise levels and cognitive development (Wachs & Gruen, 1982). Observers' ratings of overall noise levels in the home from both interior (e.g., TV, appliances) and exterior (e.g., traffic) sources were consistently related to deficits in cognitive development in boys between 6 months and 5 years of age. Less consistent effects were noted in girls. The findings have been replicated both by Wachs and other investigators (see Wachs & Gruen, 1982) and have been shown both cross-sectionally and across a 1-year time span.

Negative effects of noise on the cognitive development of older children also have been found. Kindergartners exposed to greater home noise take longer to find target stimuli from among a background of visual items during quiet conditions. They also have poorer incidental memory for nontarget items when subsequently tested on a recognition memory test (Heft, 1979). These negative effects of chronic noise hold after controlling for various sociodemographic variables. Exposure to traffic noise at school also has been associated with deficits on a measure of mental concentration among elementary school children (Karsdorf & Klappach, 1968). Unfortunately, data are not available on the comparisons of samples in this study.

Given some of the cognitive deficits found for children chronically exposed to noise, it is not surprising that several investigators have explored possible correlations between noise exposure at school and scholastic achievement. Five out of seven field studies have uncovered negative correlations between ambient noise levels and reading achievement (see Cohen et al., 1986, for a detailed summary). Several patterns are revealed in the findings.

Negative effects are stronger in the upper elementary school grades, starting at about the fifth grade. These age-related trends could be due to several factors. Children in the upper grades generally have had longer noise exposure.

Cohen, Glass, and Singer (1973), for example, have found that children exposed to traffic noise at home are significantly more affected by the noise the longer they have lived in their apartment. Alternatively, reading tests for older children may be more reliable, and thus more sensitive in measuring the harmful effects of noise.

Another pattern in the noise and achievement data is that low achievers appear more vulnerable to the harmful effects of noise (Cohen et al., 1986). In addition, levels of home noise and noise at school may interact. Children exposed to high levels of exterior noise in both locations may be more at risk for harmful cognitive effects (Cohen et al., 1986).

Interestingly, the two studies finding no effects of noise on reading achievement compared children from different schools rather than different rooms within the same school (Cohen et al., 1986; Moch-Sibony, 1984). Presumably, additional sources of variance in reading curricula, teacher training, etc., could increase the probability of Type II errors in these studies. One final piece of evidence worthy of note is that one experimenter returned to the same school after sound attenuation had been instituted and evaluated new children from the same quiet and previously noisy classrooms. Following the attenuation there were no longer significant differences in reading achievement, as there had been previously (Bronzaft & McCarthy, 1975), between children from classrooms on the side of the building close to elevated train tracks and children on the opposite side of the building (Bronzaft, 1981).

Distraction from noise may have indirect effects on cognitive development because of alterations in parents' and teachers' behaviors. Teachers in noisy schools pause when trains or airplanes pass. This may interrupt speech and reduce instruction time (Bronzaft & McCarthy, 1975; Crook & Langdon, 1974). Instructors in schools near airports also report that noise reduces their effectiveness as teachers and makes them feel more tired at the end of the day (Crook & Langdon, 1974). Of related interest, teachers in open classrooms frequently restrict certain activities because of fears about disturbing others (Ahrentzen & Evans, 1984; Gump & Good, 1976).

An important question raised by the array of negative effects of noise on cognitive development is, What is the nature of the mechanism(s) responsible for these effects? What is it about noise that produces negative outcomes in children? One reason we believe overstimulation plays some role are findings in Wachs' work (Wachs & Gruen, 1982) that children in noisy homes who have had the opportunity to escape noise by access to a stimulus shelter suffer no cognitive deficits.

Children may adapt to overstimulation by filtering out unwanted stimuli. This tuning out strategy may overgeneralize, however, such that children tune out stimuli indiscriminately. For example, chronic noise exposure is associated with deficits in auditory discrimination (Cohen et al., 1973; Moch-Sibony, 1984). Auditory discrimination tasks, measured under quiet conditions, evaluate the child's ability to distinguish between similar sounding words (e.g., boat–goat). Auditory discrimination in turn is related to reading acquisition (Cohen et al., 1973). In another study of a different noise source, Cohen and his colleagues (Cohen et al., 1986) were unable to replicate these effects but found that children chronically exposed to aircraft noise at school were less accurate in choosing the best signal-to-noise ratio among several alternatives. The decibel level of the signal (a man's voice) was constant against a background of varying white noise levels. Moreover, the longer the child had been attending the noisy school, the stronger the effect. In each of the above studies, children were tested with standard audiometric procedures and were found to have no auditory damage.

If children cope with chronic noise by filtering-out strategies, then they should be less distracted by auditory stimuli. Heft (1979) had kindergartners from quiet and noisy homes perform a figure-matching task under quiet and auditory distraction conditions. Children from the noisy homes were affected significantly less by the distraction than were their counterparts from quiet homes. Cohen and others (1986) found similar results but only for children exposed to aircraft noise at school for two years or less; with longer exposure the effect reversed.

Preschool children attending noisy daycare centers may also generalize cognitive strategies for coping with noise. Hambrick-Dixon (1986) compared preschoolers from noisy and quiet daycare centers. The noisy centers were proximate to elevated train tracks. Although there were no main effects of daycare center background noise levels or experimental conditions of noise during testing conditions, interactions were significant. Children from noisy daycare centers performed a visual coding task better under noisy experimental conditions than did their quiet daycare counterparts. The opposite pattern occurred under quiet experimental conditions.

Taken in their entirety, there is preliminary evidence suggesting that chronic exposure to noise may cause changes in children's cognitive strategies related to dealing with auditory distraction. Under certain circumstances these strategies may be detrimental.

Crowding

Studies of residential density and child development suggest crowding can increase various problem behaviors in children. These effects are most likely to occur when crowding is measured in people per room rather than when using areal measures like people per acre. Numerous studies have found increased incidence of juvenile delinquency among children from higher density homes. Although the trends in these data are consistent (Aiello, Thompson, & Baum, 1985), considerable methodological problems plague the majority of these studies (Baum & Paulus, 1987). Children from higher density homes also have more behavioral problems at school (Booth & Johnson, 1975; Murray, 1974;

Saegert, 1982). Several reasons may explain the tentative links between crowding and behavioral problems in children. Crowding may heighten tension among parents, which in turn affects how they respond to their children. Several studies have found greater family discord in high density households (Gove, Hughes, & Galle, 1979; Loo, 1980; Murray, 1974).

Parents in crowded homes also provide less supervision over their children (e.g., not knowing where their children play outside (Gove et al., 1979; Mitchell, 1971)). There is also less parental involvement with young children in high density homes (Bradley & Caldwell, 1984). Adults in crowded households also report relief when children are outside and are more apt to perceive their children as a hassle (Gove et al., 1979).

Male infants from homes with more people per room appear to have poorer cognitive development than their lower density counterparts. These effects have been demonstrated both cross-sectionally and longitudinally over a 1-year span (Wachs & Gruen, 1982). Elementary school children from higher density homes are more likely to be behind at school and have lower standardized reading scores in comparison with children from lower density homes (Murray, 1974; Saegert, 1982; Wedge & Petzing, 1970). Parents of children in crowded homes report more frequently that their children have no private places to study (Mitchell, 1971; Saegert, 1982). Particularly careful methodological and statistical controls were present in the Saegert study.

Children in crowded school and play situations evidence increased social withdrawal and solitary play activities in comparison to children in the same but lower density settings (Evans, 1978). Children also engage in less cooperative behavior immediately following high density exposure in the laboratory (Aiello et al., 1979). The data on crowding and aggression in children are more complex. Children from high density homes report greater feelings of anger, plus greater annoyance with others (Saegert, 1982). On the other hand, several school and laboratory studies yield mixed results (Evans, 1978). Some studies report increased aggression among crowded children, whereas other researchers have found either less aggression or no changes as a function of density in the classroom or laboratory. Trends in the data reveal aggression among crowded children is more likely when there are a limited number of toys to be shared (Rohe & Patterson, 1974) or when the children have pre-existing behavioral disorders (Loo, 1978).

As in the case of noise, some of these negative effects of crowding on children's behavior may be the direct results of overstimulation and interference caused by the close presence of other children or family members. It is also possible that some of the negative effects of crowding are the indirect result of efforts to adapt to chronic high density living. For example, children may withdraw from social contact as a way to cope with crowded circumstances. This strategy, like tuning out in noisy environments, may become overgeneralized.

Architectural design

Among the more important objectives of open plan schools is to expose children to a wider variety of learning opportunities. Although many open plan schools appear to achieve this objective (Ahrentzen, Jue, Skorpanich, & Evans, 1982; Gump, 1987; Weinstein, 1979), visual and auditory distraction are common complaints in these settings. Both the volume of open, undifferentiated spaces and the openness of classroom perimeters are positively correlated with visual distraction (Ahrentzen & Evans, 1984; Moore, 1987). In addition, teachers' complaints and unobtrusive observations indicate more off-task time in open classrooms when compared with more traditional designs (Gump, 1974; Gump & Good, 1976).

Evaluations of open plan classrooms architecturally modified to create better defined activity spaces with less visual and auditory distraction reveal improved utilization of space in the classroom (Weinstein, 1977), more involvement and engagement in educational activities and less passive behaviors (Moore, 1987; Weinstein, 1977), fewer classroom interruptions and nonsubstantive questions (Evans & Lovell, 1979), and more child-initiated behaviors and exploration (Moore, 1987).

Excessive stimulation in poorly designed open plan schools may also account for the desire of children in these settings to be left alone or to get away from all of the noise and stimulation (Ahrentzen et al., 1982; Gump, 1987). Perhaps this form of social withdrawal, as in crowded situations, is a coping strategy that some children employ in poorly designed open plan classrooms. Although the connection to withdrawal is speculative, children in open plan classrooms have fewer close friends in the classroom and report feeling more socially isolated at school (Hallinan, 1979). Reiss and Dydhalo (1975) have also found some evidence for the development of tuning-out strategies among children in open plan classrooms.

Summary

Cognitive development may be negatively affected by high levels of physical stimulation. Both crowding and noise cause increased distraction, which may overburden developing cognitive systems. Overcrowding also heightens family tensions, creating more stressful interpersonal interactions. Poorly designed open plan learning environments with large, undifferentiated spaces, open perimeters, and ill-defined activity boundaries lead to high levels of distraction. Children may adapt to stimulus overload by turning-out or withdrawal strategies, which in turn may have negative influences on human development.

Assessment of environmental stimulation levels has not been adequately investigated. Studies of children and the physical environment typically measure a very restricted range of setting characteristics. For example, most studies of noise compare quiet conditions to only one level of noise. Investigations with such restricted ranges may cause misspecification of an effect. As suggested by Wohlwill (1974), relations between background stimulation and outcome functions are probably curvilinear. Restricted range also reduces the power of statistical analyses to detect true effects. Further, with a narrow range of values on the environmental variable, we cannot check for possible dose–response relations (Evans & Cohen, 1987).

Additional research is also needed to understand how children perceive the physical environment. We know extremely little, for example, about whether children perceive high density homes as crowded (Aiello et al., 1985). We are also ignorant about the implications of differing perceptions. Work in open plan schools shows, for example, that teachers and elementary school students do not perceive negative environmental conditions similarly (Ahrentzen, 1980). Assessment of perceived environmental characteristics, however, raises problems of its own. As discussed by Kasl in Chapter 4, subjective measures of independent variables can create tautological arguments, often reduce methods variance, and may reflect subject characteristics such as neuroticism. On the other hand, subjective evaluations of the physical environment can strongly color outcomes, particularly those related to psychological stress reactions.

Functional Complexity

The previous section, Stimulation, described background stimuli, emphasizing the sheer amounts of stimulation impinging upon children from their physical surroundings. In contrast, functional complexity refers to characteristics of focal, environmental stimuli (Heft, 1979; Wohlwill & Heft, 1987). As seen in the previous section, some of the aversive effects of overstimulation relate to interference with focal perception. Many of the negative effects of noise on cognitive development, for example, are probably related to distraction.

Functional complexity of focal environmental stimuli for children has been examined primarily in terms of objects such as play materials. Functional complexity consists of two principle dimensions: variety and responsiveness. Variety refers to the number of different characteristics of an object. Thus a functionally complex object might consist of multiple colors, shapes, and textures. Still greater complexity would be added by an object that moves or changes in some other way. Responsiveness is the degree to which physical stimuli provide feedback to the child about the effects of his actions. When a young child manipulates an object that responds differentially to variable input, that object is responsive.

Learning and play materials

Studies in both the home and school suggest that greater variety and responsiveness of objects is associated with gains in cognitive development and more adaptive behaviors. Classrooms with more variety in instructional materials and objects are associated with positive social interactions and greater cognitive gains (Prescott, 1987). Unfortunately, most of these studies are seriously confounded with social class.

The functional complexity of playground equipment, particularly with respect to various opportunities for manipulation and as props for imaginative play, appears to be important as well (Moore, 1985; Wohlwill & Heft, 1987). Comparisons among different types of playgrounds suggest that adventure playgrounds that are typically high in functional complexity are used more and are preferred by older children because of the greater opportunities they provide for creative, imaginative play, and various building and construction activities (Hayward, Rothenberg, & Beasley, 1974; Moore, 1983).

There is a large literature on the availability and quality of children's toys and human development (see Parke, 1978; Wachs & Gruen, 1982; and Wohlwill & Heft, 1987, for reviews). We briefly describe results from two longitudinal research programs on the social and physical home environment and cognitive development. Bradley, Caldwell, and colleagues' HOME scale (Bradley & Caldwell, 1987) includes measures of the availability of age-appropriate toys. A child's exposure to age-appropriate toys is positively correlated with intelligence in children ages 6 months to 4½ years, with stronger effects noted for boys. Early experiences, between the ages of 6 months and 1 year, are at least as important as concurrent exposure to toys in predicting preschooler intelligence. Language development in both sexes is facilitated by toys, and school performance as late as first grade may be associated with contemporaneous toy availability. Throughout these cross-sectional and longitudinal studies, toy availability is either the first or second (after parental responsiveness) most important subscale out of six in predicting cognitive development.

The other major research program on home environments and child development was conducted by Wachs and his colleagues (Wachs & Gruen, 1982). This research program, which used a more middle class sample and different but related measures of home physical and social settings, also found positive effects of toy availability on development. Wachs and Gruen (1982), however, concluded that after approximately 1 year of age, it is changes in toys rather than the sheer number of different toys available that is more closely related to cognitive development. Toy changes occur either through rotation of existing toys or addition of new toys. Wachs and Gruen also noted that effects tend to be a bit stronger for girls, whereas Bradley and Caldwell (1987) reported the opposite. Both cross-sectional and prospective associations between toy variety and cognitive development were noted.

In addition to cognitive development as measured on standardized tests, toy variety also has been linked to sensorimotor skill acquisition (Yarrow, Rubinstein, & Pederson, 1975) as well as actual use and level of competence in play with toys (Clarke-Stewart, 1973). Social outcomes may also be affected by toy availability. The presence of toys reduces anxiety reactions to parental separation (Parke, 1978). Types of toys can also influence the degree of isolated versus social play (Parke, 1978).

Children as young as 3 months of age are sensitive to responsiveness in play objects. Infants can learn to manipulate a mobile that is responsive to head turns (Watson & Ramey, 1972). Of particular interest, early experience with a responsive mobile increases the infants' competence in later use of the mobile as compared with infants who have been exposed to mobiles that were not contingent upon their head turning. Wachs and his colleagues have also found associations between responsive play objects in the home and cognitive development. Results hold true for development at the time of initial measurement and for up to 1 year later for children between the ages of 1 and 2 years (Wachs & Gruen, 1982).

Summary

The variety and responsiveness of learning materials and play objects in the young child's immediate surroundings may be important in fostering cognitive development. Studies in the home in particular suggest that during the first three years of life a rich, stimulating environment that is responsive to the child's actions is associated with benefits.

Assessment of functional complexity is problematic. To date, most researchers have relied upon observer ratings of variety or responsiveness. Unfortunately, thorough analytic research on the direct measurement of functional complexity is lacking. Furthermore, there is frequent covariation of the two components of functional complexity, variety and responsiveness. This makes it difficult to isolate the individual effects of each of these components of functional complexity. Measurements of cognitive development have generally relied upon standardized instruments with good psychometric properties. On the other hand there has not always been agreement across studies with environmental effects found on one measure of cognitive development not necessarily replicating for another related measure (cf. Wachs & Gruen, 1982).

Since many of these studies on functional complexity and children's health and well-being are conducted in real world settings; random assignment of subjects to environmental conditions is impossible. Therefore, caution is necessary in drawing causal inferences about environment–health associations. In addition to social class differences (which are controlled in most studies), parents still self-select into most environmental contexts. Crowded, noisy, or polluted conditions may be correlated with other dispositional variables. For example, people more tolerant of negative physical conditions are probably over-represented in studies of environmental stressors. Those least likely to adapt have probably already moved away. Another third kind of variable that can covary with environmental characteristics is individual belief systems. For example, comparisons of open plan classrooms with more traditional designs are often confounded with educational philosophies of teachers and/or parents.

Control

Research on both young human beings and immature animals shows that very young organisms seek environmental conditions that are stimulating, challenging, and provide opportunities to exercise mastery (White, 1959). In addition, neurological and sensorimotor development are influenced by the organisms' ability to control exposure to important, critical environmental stimuli. Active, self-directed interaction with the surrounding environment during certain critical periods influences neural and sensorimotor development (Gibson, 1969; Held, 1965).

Earlier we reviewed evidence that responsive toys may foster cognitive development. The ability to control a potentially aversive toy was investigated in one study. One-year-olds were briefly exposed to a frightening mechanical toy. Half of the children could control the onset of the toy. Children with control smiled more and looked less often at their mothers for assurance. Boys but not girls with control were also less likely to cry (Gunnar-Vongnechten, 1978).

Noise

Children chronically exposed to aversive, uncontrollable environmental conditions may suffer from symptoms similar to learned helplessness (Seligman, 1975). For example, children in noisy schools make more errors on difficult puzzles (Cohen et al., 1980, 1986; Moch-Sibony, 1984). Of particular interest, they are also more likely to simply give up on difficult puzzles before the time they have been allocated has expired. Cohen and his colleagues gave third and fourth graders a series of jigsaw puzzles. Children from noisy schools in comparison with those from quiet schools, after controlling for various sociodemographic variables, failed the puzzles more often, and if they did solve them they took longer to do so. Most important, within the 4 minutes allocated to solve a puzzle, 31% of children from the noise school gave up whereas only 7% of quiet school children failed the puzzle by giving up.

These same investigators also found children from noisy schools were more willing to abrogate choice in the testing situation. At the end of the testing sessions, children were told that as a reward they could play one of several games. Children from noisy schools were significantly more likely to allow the experimenter to choose which game to play than were the children from quiet schools.

Crowding

Children chronically exposed to residential crowding may also have control-related problems. Rodin (1976) found that elementary school children from higher density apartments were less likely to choose their own reward following an operant conditioning procedure. These children were more likely to allow the experimenter to choose their reward. Saegert (1982), however, did not find any relation between home density and the likelihood of relinquishing choice to an experimenter. Rodin (1976) also exposed children of junior high age to a standard helplessness procedure and found greater susceptibility to helplessness among children from high density apartments. Helplessness was induced by the presentation of insoluble problems. Learned helplessness was measured by performance on a subsequent similar but soluble problem.

Pollutants

Edelstein (1982) found that parents and children react with strong emotional feelings to the discovery of nearby toxic waste dumps. Prominent among these reactions are feelings of powerlessness and hopelessness. Family relationships also suffer from disagreements and anxiety over how to protect family health. Baum and colleagues (Baum, Gatchell, & Schaeffer, 1983) found, in addition to self-reports of anxiety and powerlessness, physiological and performance indices of stress in parents residing near the Three Mile Island Nuclear Power Plant for as long as 2 years following the disaster.

Summary

Considerable research with adults shows that control over aversive stressors like noise significantly attenuates negative impacts (Glass & Singer, 1972; Cohen, 1980). Unfortunately, similar investigations have not been carried out with children except for the one study of control over a frightening toy. There is some evidence, however, suggesting that chronic exposure to noisy or crowded settings may cause helplessness in children. Such children show reduced motivation to sustain performance on difficult, challenging tasks.

Control is an important modifying variable that can strongly alter the effects of stress on human health and well being. One assessment issue that has not been adequately addressed in the child–environment literature is individual differences in children's beliefs about and needs for control. Children, like adults, vary in locus of control, needs for environmental control, and so on. We do not know how much these individual differences in children interact with the physical environment.

Structure and Predictability

Predictable, more orderly environments may be important for young children. Regular locations for certain activities, as well as for various objects (e.g., clothes, toys), may enable children to learn the meaning and function of objects more readily. Predictable surroundings also foster understanding of probabilistic information. For example, structured surroundings afford estimation, testing, and decision-making about future experiences. Structure also facilitates comprehension of events that unfold over time. To understand the continuity in a series of acts and to extract underlying reasons for why and how various structures go together, some structure is required (Heft, 1985).

Regular, predictable experiences in specific places facilitate the development of attachment to those places, of a sense of ownership, or at least of a sense of familiarity with them. Regularity in daily activities also promotes feelings of security, since in children it provides them with a base that can be taken for granted, thus diminishing uncertainty in daily life. By relying on certain activities to occur in specific places, children can begin to develop a sense of coherence in life—to feel that things make sense and are purposeful. Furthermore, the development of trust and close interpersonal ties may develop out of early patterns of predictability and structure provided by adult caregivers (Boyce, 1985).

The longitudinal research programs of Wachs and Gruen (1982) and Bradley and Caldwell (1987) have found positive associations between the temporal and spatial organization of the home environment and early cognitive development. These findings have been noted both cross-sectionally and longitudinally. Wachs and Gruen (1982) also suggest that early exposure to orderliness must be continued throughout early childhood for sustained effects to occur.

Noise and crowding

Both noise and crowding may influence environmental structure and predictability. Noise may interfere with children's perception of structure because it creates distraction. Sustained attention necessary to comprehend the underlying patterns in complex objects or scenes might be disrupted by the interfering effects of noise (Heft, 1985). Noise may also interfere with event perception, since the underlying contingencies between stimulus sequences may be missed because of auditory distractions.

Residential crowding makes environments less predictable and more unstructured. Predictability is reduced because of the close presence of larger numbers of other people. There is less structure because it becomes more difficult in crowded quarters to organize activities in particular locations or at particular times of the day (Heft, 1985). For example, Bradley and Caldwell (1984) found a significant, negative correlation between residential density and ratings of organization in the home.

Architectural design

Classrooms with greater physical structure may encourage a number of desirable behaviors, including intellectual development, attention to academic tasks, and compliance with teacher requests. Large, undefined areas in poorly designed open plan classrooms may contribute to some of the problems noted in these settings, such as distraction, insufficient privacy, disorganization, and unequal usage of space (Ahrentzen et al., 1982; Rivlin & Rothenberg, 1976; Weinstein, 1979).

Morrow and Weinstein (1982) were successful in increasing kindergartners' use of literature during free play times by relocating library corners to more secluded areas but keeping them visually accessible. They also added comfortable furnishings and prominently displayed reading materials. Having a more distinctive, structured, and comfortable reading area significantly increased literature use by students. Nash (1981) compared randomly arranged elementary school classrooms to planned classrooms that had distinct areas for language, math and science, sensorimotor development, and creative skills and play. The planned settings were associated with higher self-image, more advanced sensorimotor development, and better basic skills indicative of math readiness. It is unclear how much these effects result from the design itself or stem from either differences in teaching style and/or preexisting differences among the children.

Moore (1986, 1987) found that daycare centers with better spatial definition had higher levels of child-initiated behaviors. They also fostered more exploration and use of a broader range of spaces, and more involved play behaviors. Although spatial definition is a composite variable, it consists primarily of architectural features that enhance physical structure. Specifically, well-defined spatial settings have walls or partitions or use furniture to demarcate boundaries. They also include distinctive construction elements (e.g., color, texture, floor level) to indicate separateness from adjacent spaces. There is also evidence that clear separation of classroom areas from traffic patterns reduces distraction and interruptions (Evans & Lovell, 1979; Prescott, 1987).

Environmental structure also influences cognitive mapping. Children younger than 8 years of age are affected by the presence of landmarks in their cognitive representations of geographic space. Distinctive, well-placed landmarks facilitate young children's ability to orient themselves and find their way around real world settings (Evans, 1980; Heft & Wohlwill, 1987). Landmarks may also reduce egocentric responding in infants (Evans, 1980).

Summary

Structure and predictability in the early home environment, as well as in school settings, appear to be associated with enhanced cognitive development. Environmental stressors like noise and crowding may reduce environmental structure. Some of the detrimental effects of badly designed open learning environments are apparently due to lack of structure and organization of physical space.

Additional psychometric work is needed to more carefully operationalize structure and predictability. Although initial research on structure and predictability has emphasized potential negative effects from too little order, it does not necessarily follow that the more environmental organization the better. Too much structure and predictability may create overly bland, uninteresting settings devoid of discovery, challenge, or novelty.

Exploration

Obviously an important way we learn about our surroundings is through motoric exploration. Very basic perceptual processes such as depth perception are intimately tied to exploration capabilities (Gibson, 1969). Also, as noted earlier, the ability to interact instrumentally with certain key environmental stimuli during maturation may be a critical variable in neural development.

Autonomy and self-confidence may be supported by exploratory activities as well. Exploration allows one to discover new places and objects in a self-paced manner. In this sense, exploration helps children regulate environmental exposure. Exploration also facilitates modification of suboptimal surroundings. One can escape from negative stimuli (e.g., noise) if movement is possible.

Crowding and noise

Crowding and noise may indirectly influence children's environmental exploration. Children in crowded settings engage in less active and more passive play (Evans, 1978; Loo, 1978; McGrew, 1970). There is also less gross motoric movement among children in crowded rooms (Evans, 1978). Furthermore, Shapiro (1974) reported that male (but not female) preschoolers from high density homes had deficiencies in motor skill development. Children's exploration opportunities in crowded residences may also be restricted by parents or older siblings who do not want activities to be interrupted or who wish to be alone.

Exploration opportunities

The extent of exploration infants are allowed in the home has been linked to cognitive development in several studies. Typically, extent of exploration is operationalized in one of two ways. Most often exploration is equated with the amount of floor freedom, or time allowed on the floor. Exploration is also measured by the frequency of use of playpens and other barriers. During the first year of life, greater floor freedom is positively correlated with cognitive development (Ainsworth & Bell, 1974; Beckwith, Cohen, Kopp, Parmelee, & Marcy, 1976) and with sophistication of toy play (Jennings, Harmon, Morgan, Gaiter, & Yarrow, 1979). In the second year of life, male toddlers with greater opportunity to explore the home evidence better object permanence (Wachs & Gruen, 1982). Evidence for the effects of early exploration opportunities on later cognitive development are more mixed (Wachs & Gruen, 1982).

Individual differences in the child's motoric ability to move around the immediate environment are also associated with intellectual development. Several studies indicate that self-directed exploration results in better knowledge of the spatial layout of a place. For example, young infants of the same age, but with variable mobility skills (no means of independent locomotion, movement possible in a walker, crawling ability) differ in the extent to which they rely on egocentric (i.e., body position) versus external, fixed points of reference (i.e., physical landmarks in space) to orient in a place. Infants with no locomotion experience rely almost exclusively on egocentric cues when making direction judgments. Similar trends have been found in experimental studies with toddlers who were either carried or encouraged to crawl across a space to retrieve an object previously experienced from a 180 degree perspective (Acredolo, 1988).

Among older, preschool-aged children, active exploration both of full-scale environments and of scale models yields superior acquisition of environmental cognition knowledge in comparison with passively experienced spaces or models (Evans, 1980; Heft & Wohlwill, 1987).

Opportunity to explore the outdoor environment has been linked to children's cognitive wayfinding and orientation abilities. For example, the size and accuracy of children's cognitive maps of their neighborhoods are correlated with the extent of home range allowed the child (Evans, 1980; Hart, 1979; Heft & Wohlwill, 1987). Home range is usually measured by the size of the area the child is typically allowed to play in outside the immediate grounds of the residence. As noted by Evans (1980), many of the gender differences found in children's and adolescents' cognitive mapping abilities may be attributable to parental restrictions on the home range of girls in some cultures.

Greater freedom to explore outdoor settings also broadens learning opportunities. Children with a wider home range are exposed to a greater variety of activities and behavior settings (van Vliet, 1985). Perhaps one of the major developmental milestones occurs when children are allowed to play outside the immediate home environment. The transition from the home to the street and neighborhood represents a significant increase in environmental demands, complexities, and learning opportunities placed on the child. There is a greater diversity of stimulation, more novel and challenging stimuli (e.g., traffic), plus a wider array of persons to interact with (Proshansky & Fabian, 1987).

Summary

Opportunities for exploration, initially in the home and later in the surrounding environs, may influence cognitive development and subsequently more general knowledge and understanding of the surrounding environment. Exploration opportunities are strongly tied to parental behaviors and attitudes. Perhaps parents who provide functionally complex objects, regulate exploration activities, support the use of stimulus shelters, etc., are more intelligent, progressive, and less anxious. Caution is warranted in assuming that all the effects associated with physical characteristics of the environment are caused solely by inanimate properties.

INTERRELATIONS OF ENVIRONMENTAL CHARACTERISTICS

The six environmental characteristics—pathogenic conditions, stimulation levels, functional complexity, control, structure and predictability, and exploration opportunities—have been described for the most part as single, isolated dimensions. In daily life, most of these characteristics of the physical environment are interrelated. Direct pathological effects may influence the capacity of the neural system to respond to stimulation levels. Toxins could interfere with cognitive skills so that several other aspects of a child's environmental functioning might be impaired. For example, children's ability to exercise control over the physical environment would be impaired if sensory motor dysfunction was caused by toxic exposure. Similarly, certain coping strategies might not be available to children with impaired cognitive function.

Stimulation levels and functional complexity interact in several respects. One of the primary reasons overstimulation is dysfunctional is because of distraction. Background stimuli can interfere with attention to focal properties. In particular, when sustained attention is needed to comprehend the meaning and function of objects or spaces, the distracting effects of background stimuli may be particularly disruptive. Overstimulation can also disrupt learning about sequences of stimuli that form events.

Stimulus overload resulting from overcrowding also affects access to variety of objects, since as the number of people sharing a setting goes up, the variety of available objects per person decreases (Heft, 1985). Crowding can indirectly reduce the responsiveness of an environment since with social withdrawal children and adults will have less contact with one another. The critical need for responsive parenting in infancy and early childhood may be disrupted by social withdrawal in response to high density. Crowding may also affect play behaviors by reducing active exploration and use of the environment. Parents in crowded or noisy environments may also restrict play behaviors and movement in order to reduce activity levels or to avoid disturbing neighbors. Similar restrictions on children's behaviors have been found in poorly designed, open plan classrooms.

A surfeit of information can also make settings less predictable and unstructured. Crowded settings, for example, are less predictable because of more social encounters. They are also more difficult to organize because of greater competing demands for coordination.

Variety and responsiveness in the environment reinforce exploration and dynamic interaction with surroundings. Functional complexity also supports the development of autonomy, since the child has greater opportunity to interact with the environment and receive feedback about his or her behavior. Practice in using the environment may also increase ability to exercise control, plus support more instrumental coping strategies. Conceivably, children who have more early experiences of competent interactions with their physical environments may be less susceptible to the induction of helplessness when control is difficult or impossible to exercise.

Control interacts with several of the environmental characteristics we have discussed. Control over stressors like crowding or noise reduces some of their negative effects. Control over space in the form of privacy or access to stimulus shelter may directly reduce the amount of stimulation children come into contact with. Control may also assist the child in balancing the ratio of background to focal stimulation in a setting. With control, one may be able to directly intervene to reduce background distraction or increase the saliency of focal properties.

Exploration significantly increases the child's autonomy with respect to the physical environment. It allows him or her to escape from or avoid aversive conditions, as well as to approach and learn more about a wider variety of positive environmental qualities. Thus exploration can increase the variety of focal stimuli encountered and also increase the opportunities for dynamic interactions with responsive components of settings. Children's wider access to surroundings can also increase the number of chances available to exercise direct control and autonomy over the environment itself and indirect control vis-à-vis the parents. With mobility, one can better regulate environmental experiences and do more for oneself.

Increased helplessness induced by chronic exposure to uncontrollable, aversive environmental conditions weakens the child's ability to exercise control even when it is available to him or her. Such children may be less willing to actively engage their surroundings and are perhaps more cautious and reticent to explore. Moreover, the fatigue produced by efforts to cope with environmental demands may have residual effects on performance or motivation that make it more difficult to cope with subsequent environmental insults.

CONCEPTUAL ISSUES

Several general conceptual issues are raised by our analysis of child–environment interactions. First, there is a notable absence of developmental comparisons in many studies of children and the physical environment. The absence of careful age comparisons leaves us with little systematic evidence about how children's interactions with the physical environment change with maturation. Certain physical conditions affect children at one age but not another. For example, exposure to toxic materials in utero can have deleterious effects that are not seen when exposure occurs after birth (Fein et al., 1983).

Important conceptual questions are also highlighted by attention to age as a variable in the person–environment transaction. For example, are younger children more vulnerable in general to negative environmental conditions? One could argue, for example, that younger children have less control over their environments, their coping repertoires are less developed, and their adaptive capacities may be more easily strained. In addition, some developing tissue may be more susceptible to toxic effects than are more mature structures.

Age also touches on another important conceptual issue. The role of the child's own actions in affecting the person–environment interaction has not been adequately appreciated or understood (White, 1959; Wohlwill, 1983; Wohlwill & Heft, 1987). Children actively seek out and interact with their surroundings; they are not simply passive vessels receiving stimulus input. Developing sensory and motor capacities, as well as maturing cognitive skills, significantly alter how children act upon their surroundings.

The physical environment has both direct and indirect effects on children's health and well-being. A central moderating effect of the physical environment on children is the influence of the parents (Parke, 1978). Most directly, parents can modify settings, which in turn can affect the child. The provision of certain types of toys or allowance of greater freedom to explore the environment are prominent examples. Adults may also modify their environments to better suit their own needs in ways that influence child behaviors. For example, in schools, carpeting is more comfortable than hard surfaces and reduces noise; at the same time, this prevents activities such as water play (Weinstein, 1987). Alternatively, the physical environment can influence parents' behaviors, which in turn can affect how the child is treated. If parents react with irritation or anger to living in a crowded apartment, this may influence how patient they are with their children. Social withdrawal as a coping strategy under crowded living conditions could profoundly change family interpersonal relationships.

Another type of indirect effect of environmental conditions is illustrated by cross-setting interactions. For example, noise levels at home may bear upon the child's reactions to noise at school (Cohen et al., 1986). The total amount of demands that impinge upon an individual child may also influence responses to the environment. A recent stressful life event (e.g., parental separation, starting in a new school) or relatively minor but persistent strains or hassles (e.g., long bus ride to school) may alter the vulnerability of the child to various environmental stressors.

Coping with environmental stressors like noise and crowding may have negative side-effects such as tuning out, social withdrawal, or helplessness. More study is needed on how the efforts children make to cope with aversive physical conditions influence direct environmental impacts. We also need to examine whether the coping processes in and of themselves cause harm (Cohen et al., 1986; Schönpflug, 1986).

There is a growing body of literature on the stress and coping process among children (Compas, 1987; Rutter, 1981). Most of this research focuses on psychosocial sources of stress in the family and at school. The small but intensive study of resilient children reveals various personal and situational variables that contribute to the development of persons who deal more effectively with stress. Early experiences of managing environmental stimuli and dealing with discomfort, coupled with the ability to elicit social interaction, appear to be important precursors to the development of resilience in the growing child (Garmezy, 1983; Murphy & Moriarity, 1976; Werner & Smith, 1982). The interplay of some of these factors with the physical environment has not been studied. For example, how might a crowded home environment with few opportunities for privacy and greater social withdrawal of family members from one another affect independence or social interaction skills?

Good problem-solving skills facilitate adaptive coping. Early experience and practice in managing environmental demands may help a child develop a more sophisticated problem-solving repertoire. At home this might occur through learning how to manipulate the immediate environment to avoid aversive stimuli or to tap into more desirable sources of information. At school or on the playground, opportunities to engage one's curiosity; to play in increasingly complex, challenging games; and to discover new objects and places might support the development of problem-solving skills.

Resilience is also encouraged by early freedom to explore the environment. Physical barriers that prevent exploration or parenting practices that discourage it could interfere with the development of resilience. Housing design at both the micro and macro level can influence exploration. Parental concerns about stairways, proximity to heavy traffic, and high rise buildings are all associated with parental restrictions on exploration.

The structure and predictability of one's early physical surroundings might facilitate the development of planning skills. The tendency of children to exercise foresight and take active steps to deal with environmental challenges may increase in circumstances where children can make sense out of their surroundings (Kaplan & Kaplan, 1982).

Individual differences in genetic constitution, physiological readiness, coping processes, and psychosocial factors in the child's environment, all may moderate how a particular child reacts to the physical environment. Therefore, if we only examine main effects of environmental conditions on children's health and well-being, small or insignificant effects may obscure important subgroups of the child population who are at risk (Fein et al., 1983; Wachs & Gruen, 1982).

PROMOTING HEALTHY DEVELOPMENT

We want environments for children that foster security, trust, and the development of personal identity and competence. Settings need to provide opportunities for exploration; they need to be interesting, challenging, and malleable. Children also require a range of social opportunities, from solitude to broad contact with groups of heterogeneous people (David & Weinstein, 1987). In addition, contact with environmental hazards and crowded or noisy environments should be avoided. Although there is little hard data on how the physical environment can promote healthy development, some speculations are warranted from the analysis we have provided.

Obviously, exposure to environmental hazards should be minimized, particularly during gestation and early infancy. Young organisms appear especially vulnerable to harmful effects from pollutants, heavy metals, various solvents, and other chemical compounds. Given the paucity of data on behavioral effects of chemicals and the exponential growth of new compounds introduced into the environment annually, more vigilance is critically needed.

Stimulation levels, particularly during infancy, should be kept moderately low. Infants do not adapt well to sudden or large changes in stimulation. Preschoolers should be exposed to more stimulation but given opportunities to escape from or modify the stimuli they encounter. Crowding and noise can adversely affect cognitive functioning, social relationships, and the development of self efficacy in young children. The importance of refuge from overstimulation has been noted in overcrowded homes, noisy residences, and inadequately designed classrooms. On the other hand, children raised in isolation do not fare well either. Instead, homes and communities need to provide a gradient of social and physical stimulation. See Zimring (1982) for a discussion of how residences and neighborhoods can be designed to support gradients of stimulation.

Preschoolers and elementary school children need increasingly complex, responsive focal features in their environments. Various objects and toys can provide practice in acting upon the environment and receiving feedback about those actions. It is likely that the availability of functionally complex objects, coupled with the freedom to explore the immediate environment, promotes healthy development in young children.

Young children need predictability and structure in their surroundings. Learning to associate certain people and places with specific activities and functions may be a prerequisite for the development of trust and security. Environmental coherence also affords better comprehension about where things are and what they do.

Preschool and elementary school children spend considerable amounts of time in institutionalized settings, including daycare, school, and health care facilities. Typically, institutional environments emphasize uniformity and control. Greater efforts should be made to change the physical contexts of institutions to minimize surveillance, regimentation, and the overly public qualities they often embody (Rivlin & Wolfe, 1985).

Settings for early learning should offer a variety of learning centers that are easily accessible—open enough for the child to see learning opportunities but with sufficient closure to shield auditory and visual distraction. Activity areas should be well defined with clear boundaries, separate from pathways, and large enough to minimize crowding and interference but not so large that unused or dead spaces occur.

The size of functioning units may be a critical variable for children. Larger families, larger classrooms, larger daycare centers, and larger housing complexes have all been associated with potential difficulties for children. The amount of resources available, the quality of parental or adult caregiver interaction, and the extent of social and play opportunities can all be adversely affected by large size (Wicker, 1983).

Experiences of autonomy and mastering environmental demands may be critical precursors to the development of the kind of good problem-solving skills that underlie competent living in the modern world. The availability of objects and spaces of proper scale so that young children can use them; the provision of responsive objects; and access to functionally complex and challenging play spaces may all promote early experiences of environmental mastery (Weinstein, 1987). Practice at managing surroundings also teaches children how to cope with adverse, environmental demands. It may also gird them against adverse consequences from exposure to uncontrollable events. Conversely, early experiences with aversive, uncontrollable environmental conditions may increase vulnerability to feelings of helplessness. Studies of resilient children reveal that early experiences of manageable environmental challenges, responsive and supportive parenting, and fostering of independence and self-efficacy are all associated with the development of children who are more effective in managing environmental demands.

REFERENCES

Acredolo, L. P. (1988). Infant mobility and spatial development. In J. Stiles-Davis, M. Kritchevsky, & U. Bellugi (Eds.), *Spatial Cognition: Brain Bases and Development* (pp. 157–186). Hillsdale, NJ: Erlbaum.

Ahrentzen, S. (1980). *Environment-behavior relations in the classroom setting: A multi modal research perspective.* Unpublished masters' thesis, University of California, Irvine.

Ahrentzen, S., & Evans, G. W. (1984). Distraction, privacy, and classroom design. *Environment and Behavior, 16,* 437–454.

Ahrentzen, S., Jue, G., Skorpanich, M. A., & Evans, G. W. (1982). School environments and stress. In G. W. Evans (Ed.), *Environmental stress* (pp. 224–255). New York: Cambridge.

Aiello, J., Nicosia, G., & Thompson, D. E. (1979). Physiological, social, and behavioral consequences of crowding on children and adolescents. *Child Development, 50,* 195–202.

Aiello, J. R., Thompson, D. E., & Baum, A. (1985). Children, crowding, and control: Effects of environmental stress on social behavior. In J. F. Wohlwill & W. van Vliet (Eds.), *Habitats for children* (pp. 97–124). Hillsdale, NJ: Erlbaum.

Ainsworth, M., & Bell, S. (1974). Mother infant interaction and the development of competence. In K. Connolly & J. S. Bruner (Eds.), *The growth of competence* (pp. 97–118). New York: Academic.

Baum, A., Gatchell, R., & Schaeffer, M. (1983). Emotional, behavioral, and physiological effects of chronic stress at Three Mile Island. *Journal of Consulting and Clinical Psychology, 51,* 565–572.

Baum, A., & Paulus, P. B. (1987). Crowding. In D. Stokols & I. Altman (Eds.), *Handbook of environmental psychology* (pp. 533–570). New York: Wiley.

Beckwith, L., Cohen, S., Kopp, C., Parmelee, A., & Marcy, J. (1976). Caregiver–infant interaction and early cognitive development. *Child Development, 47,* 579–587.

Berglund, B., & Lindvall, T. (1986). Sensory reactions to sick buildings. *Environment International, 12,* 147–159.

Booth, A., & Johnson, D. (1975). The effect of crowding on child health and development. *American Behavioral Scientist, 18,* 736–750.

Boyce, W. T. (1985). Social support, family relations, and children. In S. Cohen & S. L. Syme (Eds.), *Social support and health* (pp. 151–173). New York: Academic Press.

Bradley, R., & Caldwell, B. (1984). The HOME inventory and family demographics. *Development Psychology, 20,* 315–320.

Bradley, R., & Caldwell, M. (1987). Early environment and cognitive competence: The Little Rock study. *Early Child Development and Care, 27,* 307–341.

Bronzaft, A. (1981). The effect of a noise abatement program on reading ability. *Journal of Environmental Psychology, 3,* 215–222.

Bronzaft, A., & McCarthy, D (1975). The effect of elevated train noise on reading ability. *Environment and Behavior, 7,* 517–527.

Byers, R. K., & Lord, E. E. (1943). Late effects of lead poisoning on mental development. *American Journal of Diseases of Children, 66,* 471–494.

Clarke-Stewart, K. A. (1973). Interactions between mothers and their young children: Characteristics and consequences. *Monographs of the Society for Research in Child Development, 38,* (6-7, Serial No. 153).

Cohen, S. (1980). Aftereffects of stress on human performance and social behavior: A review of research and theory. *Psychological Bulletin, 88,* 82–108.

Cohen, S., Evans, G. W., Krantz, D. S., & Stokols, D. (1980). Physiological, motivational, and cognitive effects of aircraft noise on children: Moving from the laboratory to the field. *American Psychologist, 35,* 231–243.

Cohen, S., Evans, G. W., Krantz, D. S., Stokols, D., & Kelly, S. (1982). Aircraft noise and children: Longitudinal and cross-sectional evidence on adaptation to noise and the effectiveness of noise abatement. *Journal of Personality and Social Psychology, 40,* 331–345.

Cohen, S., Evans, G. W., Stokols, D., & Krantz, D. S. (1986). *Behavior, health, and environmental stress.* New York: Plenum.

Cohen, S., Glass, D. C., & Singer, J. E. (1973). Apartment noise, auditory discrimination, and reading ability in children. *Journal of Experimental Social Psychology, 9,* 407–422.

Compas, B. E. (1987). Coping with stress during childhood and adolescence. *Psychological Bulletin, 101,* 393–403.

Crook, M., & Langdon, F. (1974). The effects of aircraft noise in schools around London airport. *Journal of Sound and Vibration, 34,* 221–232.

David, T. G., & Weinstein, C. S. (1987). The built environment and children's development. In C. S. Weinstein & T. G. David (Eds.), *Spaces for children* (pp. 3–18). New York: Plenum.

Edelstein, M. R. (1982). Contaminated children: Exposure in Jackson, New Jersey. *Childhood City Quarterly, 9,* 19–32.

Evans, G. W. (1978). Crowding and the developmental process. In A. Baum & Y. Epstein (Eds.), *Human response to crowding* (pp. 117–139). Hillsdale, NJ: Erlbaum.

Evans, G. W. (1980). Environmental cognition. *Psychological Bulletin, 88,* 259–287.

Evans, G. W., & Cohen, S. (1987). Environmental stress. In D. Stokols & I. Altman (Eds.), *Handbook of environmental psychology* (pp. 571–610). New York: Wiley.

Evans, G. W., & Lovell, B. (1979). Design modification in an open-plan school. *Journal of Educational Psychology, 71,* 41–49.

Evans, G. W., & Tafalla, R. (1987). Measurement of environmental annoyance. In H. Koelga (Ed.), *Environmental annoyance: Characterization, measurement, and control* (pp. 11–28). Amsterdam: Elsevier.

Fein, G., Schwartz, P., Jacobson, S., & Jackson, J. (1983). Environmental toxins and behavioral development. *American Psychologist, 38,* 1188–1197.

Garmezy, N. (1983). Stressors of childhood. In N. Garmezy & M. Rutter (Eds.), *Stress, coping, and development in children* (pp. 43–84). New York: McGraw-Hill.

Gibson, E. J. (1969). *Principles of perceptual learning and development.* New York: Appleton-Century-Crofts.

Glass, D. C., & Singer, J. E. (1972). *Urban stress.* New York: Academic.

Gove, W. R., Hughes, M., & Galle, V. (1979). Overcrowding in the home: An empirical investigation of its possible pathological consequences. *American Sociological Review, 44,* 59–80.

Gump, P. (1974). Operating environments in open and traditional schools. *School Review, 84,* 575–593.

Gump, P. (1987). School and classroom environments. In D. Stokols & I. Altman (Eds.), *Handbook of environmental psychology* (pp. 691–732). New York: Wiley.

Gump, P., & Good, L. (1976). Environments operating in open space and traditionally designed schools. *Journal of Architectural Research, 5,* 20–27.

Gunnar-Vongnechten, M. (1978). Changing a frightening toy into a pleasant toy by allowing the infant to control its actions. *Developmental Psychology, 14,* 157–162.

Hallinan, M. T. (1979). Structural effects on children's friendships and cliques. *Social Psychology Quarterly, 42*(1), 43–54.

Hambrick-Dixon, P. J. (1986). Effects of experimentally imposed noise on task performance of black children attending day care centers near elevated subway trains. *Developmental Psychology, 22,* 259–264.

Hart, R. (1979). *Children's experience of place.* New York: Irvington.

Hayward, D. G., Rothenberg, M., & Beasley, R. (1974). Children's play and urban playground environments: A comparison of traditional, contemporary, and adventure playground types. *Environment and Behavior, 6,* 131–168.

Hebb, D. O. (1949). *The organization of behavior.* New York: Wiley.

Heft, H. (1979). Background and focal environmental conditions of the home and attention in young children. *Journal of Applied Social Psychology, 9,* 47–69.

Heft, H. (1985). High residential density and perceptual-cognitive development: An examination of the effects of crowding and noise in the home. In J. F. Wohlwill & W. van Vliet (Eds.), *Habitats for children* (pp. 39–75). Hillsdale, NJ: Erlbaum.

Heft, H., & Wohlwill, J. F. (1987). Environmental cognition in children. In D. Stokols & I. Altman (Eds.), *Handbook of environmental psychology* (pp. 175–204). New York: Wiley.

Held, R. (1965). Plasticity in sensory-motor systems. *Scientific American, 213,* 84–94.

Jacobson, J. L., Jacobson, S. W., Fein, G., Schwartz, P., & Dowler, J. (1984). Prenatal exposure to an environmental toxin: A test of the multiple effects model. *Developmental Psychology, 20,* 523–532.

Jennings, K., Harmon, R., Morgan, G., Gaiter, J., & Yarrow, L. (1979). Exploratory play as an index of mastery motivation: Relationships to persistence, cognitive functioning, and environmental measures. *Developmental Psychology, 15,* 386–394.

Kaplan, S., & Kaplan, R. (1982). *Cognition and environment.* New York: Praeger.

Karagodina, I., Soldatkina, S., Vinokur, I., & Klimukhin, A. (1969). Effect of aircraft noise on the population near airports. *Hygiene and Sanitation, 34,* 182–187.

Karsdorf, G., & Klappach, H. (1968). The influence of traffic noise on the health and performance of secondary school students in a large city. *Zeitschrift fur die Gesamte Hygiene, 14,* 52–54.

Loo, C. M. (1978). Density, crowding, and preschool children. In A. Baum & Y. Epstein (Eds.), *Human response to crowding* (pp. 371–388). Hillsdale, NJ: Erlbaum.

Loo, C. M. (1980). *Chinatown: Crowding and mental health.* Montreal: American Psychological Association.

McGrew, P. L. (1970). Social and spatial density effects of spacing behavior in preschool children. *Journal of Child Psychology and Psychiatry, 11,* 197–205.

Mitchell, R. (1971). Some social implications of high density housing. *American Sociological Review, 36,* 18–29.

Moch-Sibony, A. (1984). Study of the effects of noise on the personality and certain psychomotor and intellectual aspects of children, after a prolonged exposure. *Travail Humane, 47,* 155–165.

Moore, G. T. (1983). *Some effects of physical and social environmental variables on children's behavior: Two studies of children's outdoor play and child care environments.* Unpublished doctoral dissertation, Clark University, Worcester, MA.

Moore, G. T. (1985). State of the art in play environment research and applications. In J. Frost (Ed.), *When children play* (pp. 171–192). Wheaton, MD: Association for Child Education International.

Moore, G. T. (1986). Effects of the spatial definition of behavior settings on children's behavior: A quasi-experimental field study. *Journal of Environmental Psychology, 6,* 205–231.

Moore, G. T. (1987). The physical environment and cognitive development in child care centers. In C. S. Weinstein & T. G. David (Eds.), *Spaces for children: The built environment and child development* (pp. 41–72). New York: Plenum.

Morrow, L., & Weinstein, C. S. (1982). Increasing children's use of literature through program and physical design changes. *Elementary School Journal, 83,* 131–137.

Murphy, L. B., & Moriarity, A. (1976). *Vulnerability, coping, and growth.* New Haven, CT: Yale University Press.

Murray, R. (1974). The influence of crowding on children's behavior. In D. Canter & T. Lee (Eds.), *Psychology and the built environment* (pp. 112–117).

Nash, C. (1981). The effects of classroom spatial organization on four and five year old children's learning. *British Journal of Psychology, 51,* 144–155.

National Academy of Sciences. (1986). *Environmental tobacco smoke.* Washington, DC: NAS Press.

Needleman, H. L., Gunnoe, C., Leviton, A., Reed, R., Peresie, H., Maker, C., & Barrett, P. (1979). Deficits in psychologic and classroom performance of children with elevated dentine lead levels. *New England Journal of Medicine, 300,* 59–65.

Parke, R. D. (1978). Children's home environments: Social and cognitive effects. In J. F. Wohlwill and I. Altman (Eds.), *Children and the environment* (pp. 33–81). New York: Plenum.

Prescott, E. (1987). The environment as organizer of intent in child-care settings. In C. S. Weinstein & T. G. David (Eds.), *Spaces for children* (pp. 73–88). New York: Plenum.

Proshansky, H. M., & Fabian, A. (1987). The development of place identity in the child. In C. S. Weinstein & T. G. David (Eds.), *Spaces for children* (pp. 21–40). New York: Plenum.

Reiss, S., & Dydhalo, N. (1975). Persistence, achievement, and open space environments. *Journal of Educational Psychology, 67,* 506–513.

Rivlin, L. G., & Rothenberg, M. (1976). The use of space in open classrooms. In H. M. Proshansky, W. H. Ittelson, & L. G. Rivlin (Eds.), *Environmental psychology: People and their physical settings* (2nd ed., pp. 479–489). New York: Holt, Rinehart, & Winston.

Rivlin, L. G., & Wolfe, M. (1985). *Institutional settings in children's lives.* New York: Wiley.

Rodin, J. (1976). Density, perceived choice and response to controllable and uncontrollable outcomes. *Journal of Experimental Social Psychology, 12,* 564–578.

Rohe, W., & Patterson, A. H. (1974). *The effects of varied levels of resources and density on behavior in a day care center.* Milwaukee, WI: Environmental Design Research Association.

Rutter, M. (1980). Raised lead levels and impaired cognitive/behavioral functioning: A review of the evidence. *Developmental Medicine and Child Neurology, 22,* 1–26.

Rutter, M. (1981). Stress, coping, and development: Some issues and some questions. *Journal of Child Psychology and Psychiatry, 22,* 323–356.

Saegert, S. (1982). Environment and children's mental health: Residential density and low income children. In A. Baum & J. E. Singer (Eds.), *Handbook of psychology and health* (pp. 247–271). Hillsdale, NJ: Erlbaum.

Schönpflug, W. (1986). Behavior economics as an approach to stress theory. In M. Appley & R. Trumbull (Eds.), *Dynamics of stress* (pp. 81–98). New York: Plenum.

Seligman, M. E. P. (1975). *Helplessness: On depression, development and death.* San Francisco: Freeman.

Shapiro, A. (1974). Effect of family density and mother's education on preschooler's motor skills. *Perceptual and Motor Skills, 38,* 79–86.

Thompson, W., & Grusec, J. (1970). Studies of early experience. In P. H. Mussen (Ed.), *Carmichael's manual of child psychology* (3rd ed., pp. 565–654). New York: Wiley.

van Vliet, W. (1985). The role of housing type, household density, and neighborhood density in peer interaction and social adjustment. In J.F. Wohlwill

& W. van Vliet (Eds.), *Habitats for children* (pp. 165–200). Hillsdale, NJ: Erlbaum.

Wachs, T. D., & Gruen, G. E. (1982). *Early experience and human development.* New York: Plenum.

Watson, J., & Ramey, C. (1972). Reactions to response-contingent stimulation in early infancy. *Merrill Palmer Quarterly, 18,* 219–228.

Wedge, P., & Petzing, J. (1970). Housing for children. *Housing Review, 19,* 165–166.

Weinstein, C. S. (1977). Modifying student behavior in an open classroom through changes in the physical design. *American Education Research Journal, 14,* 249–262.

Weinstein, C. S. (1979). The physical environment of the school: A review of the research. *Review of Educational Research, 49,* 577–610.

Weinstein, C. S. (1987). Designing preschool classrooms to support development. In C. S. Weinstein & T. David (Eds.), *Spaces for children* (pp. 159–186). New York: Plenum.

Weinstein, C. S., & David, T. G. (Eds.). (1987). *Spaces for children.* New York: Plenum.

Weiss, B. (1983). Behavioral toxicology and environmental health science. *American Psychologist, 38,* 1174–1187.

Werner, E. E., & Smith, R. S. (1982). *Vulnerable but invincible: A study of resilient children.* New York: McGraw-Hill.

White, R. W. (1959). Motivation reconsidered: The concept of competence. *Psychological Review, 66,* 297–333.

Wicker, A. (1983). *An introduction to ecological psychology.* New York: Cambridge University Press.

Wohlwill, J. F. (1974). Human adaptation to levels of environmental stimulation. *Human Ecology, 2,* 1–27.

Wohlwill, J. F. (1983). The physical and the social environment as factors in development. In D. Magnusson & V. P. Allen (Eds.), *Human development: An interactional perspective* (pp. 111–129). New York: Academic.

Wohlwill, J. F., & Heft, H. (1987). The physical environment and the development of the child. In D. Stokols & I. Altman (Eds.), *Handbook of environmental psychology* (pp. 281–328). New York: Wiley.

Yarrow, L., Rubinstein, J., & Pederson, F. (1975). *Infant and environment: Early cognitive and motivational development.* New York: Halsted.

Zimring, C. (1982). The built environment as a source of psychological stress: Impacts of buildings and cities on satisfaction and behavior. In G. W. Evans (Ed.), *Environmental stress* (pp. 151–178). New York: Cambridge University Press.

6

COMMUNITY NEEDS ASSESSMENT

Jean E. Rhodes

University of Illinois at Urbana-Champaign

Leonard A. Jason

DePaul University

Community needs assessment is a process used to determine the extent and kinds of needs that are in a community, to evaluate existing resources, and to provide information for planning new service programs based on the community needs, interest, and limited resources (Siegel, Attkisson, & Cohn, 1977). In addition, needs assessment strategies are useful in specifying resources that can be channeled to respond to unmet needs, and in defining the social, environmental, and biological etiology of certain conditions, eventually leading to more effective services (Siegel, Attkisson, & Carson, 1978). Indeed, Baker (1974) argued that no rational human service can be created in the absence of such assessment and definition.

Community services may be targeted to a wide array of populations and concerns, and it is beyond the scope of this work to address the specific issues involved in needs assessment procedures applicable to the full range of potential target populations. Rather, we will endeavor to provide a brief overview of the needs assessment procedures and conceptual issues as they are related to community-based health promotion programs. To accomplish this goal, we first present some of the applications, advantages, and disadvantages of the most common methods of needs assessment, including (a) the community forum, (b) social indicator analysis, (c) the field survey, and (d) key informants. The actual use and selection of these approaches is carefully discussed elsewhere (Cox, Carmichael, & Dightman, 1979; Warheit, Bell, & Schwab, 1977; Zautra & Simons, 1978). We devote the remainder of the chapter to addressing some of the conceptual issues inherent to the process of community needs assessment. It is suggested that the selection and use of these techniques reflect certain values and biases concerning the importance of, etiology of, and solutions to community health disorders. We further argue that needs assessments are often conducted in the absence of the careful and open consideration of such values. Ecologically valid strategies that emphasize the explication of values, empowerment, and collaboration are presented.

NEEDS ASSESSMENT STRATEGIES

Community Forums

One of the most commonly used methods of assessing the need for community services is the community forum. This approach typically consists of public meetings during which community members express their beliefs regarding the need for differing types of programs. Questionnaires may be distributed for community members to rank-order the community's needs as they perceive them. More frequently, the data are gathered less formally through an open dialogue. Planners then compile this information, assess a community's needs, and evaluate extant programs in the context of those needs (Warheit, Vega, & Buhl-Auth, 1983).

Throughout this process, the community members may develop a greater awareness of available services, and the agency that has sponsored the forum is likely to become more visible and appreciated in the community. Despite these benefits, there are a number of difficulties that limit the validity and utility of the community needs assessment approach. Community members with serious social and health needs often do not or cannot attend public meetings. Adding to this situation is the tendency for forums to be dominated by organized groups that have the capacity to control meetings through their systematic organization and spokespersons. Another limitation is that the forum may increase expectations on the part of the residents regarding the development of programs that the conducting agency may not be able to address.

Additionally, community residents often do not know of the problems, either because they do not have access to some of the facts or because they are unaware of certain subtle contingencies that strongly affect their community. For example, Jason and Liotta (1982) found that jaywalking occurred at a busy intersection at very high rates (38%) if pedestrians walked in a counterclockwise direction, but only at 2% if they walked in a clockwise direction. This is important because thousands of pedestrians are killed or injured while jaywalking each year. In this study, the differential findings were due to the fact that the timing of walk and no-walk light sequences was very different in the clockwise and counterclockwise directions. When questioned, the public was unaware of these differential contingencies. Community assessors can see as their role documenting contingencies or influences that shape the behavior of community residents.

Rates-under-treatment

A second widely used method of community assessment is the rates-under-treatment approach. This approach relies on a descriptive list of the clients utilizing the services of an agency. The basic assumption underlying this method is that those who receive care represent the population in need. Unfortunately, research evidence clearly indicates that many persons in serious need of mental health services do not receive them. Beyond this chief concern, utilization rates are less helpful in assessing needs for health promotion/prevention services, since these utilization rates represent manifestations of a problem that has already developed (Warheit et al., 1983).

Social and Health Indictor Analysis

Another frequently utilized needs assessment strategy for planners of community-based health promotion services is social indicators analysis. The underlying assumption of the approach is that estimates of needs and social well-being of those in a community can be made by examining selected social and demographic descriptors that have been found to correlate highly with service utilization (e.g., race, socioeconomic status, community stability) (Siegel et al., 1978). Such data are derived from community surveys, social and/or health agencies, census records, health departments, universities, publications, and clearinghouses.

The social indicator technique may be particularly helpful in identifying and ultimately strengthening groups of individuals at high risk for the development of social or health problems (Cox et al., 1979; Felner & Aber, 1983). Unlike other assessment procedures discussed above, this approach does not require direct reports of perceived need or problems. A notable limitation of this approach is its dependence on the community members' needs being identified by others. Given the potential biases associated with this process, it may be insufficient to depend on the planners to be both sensitive and oriented to attend to the needs of community members who are not showing obvious health or behavioral problems. Even when identified, data often reflect the number of times a problem is reported rather than the actual incidence of the problem. For example, the number of reported drunk driving or domestic violence arrests is likely to be far lower than the actual incidence of these problems. In addition, because data tend to be collected for larger geographic areas, the data that are available may not pertain to smaller communities or rural areas of interest. Related to this problem is the fact that different data collection agencies tend to subdivide data by different areas. For example, the district boundaries of the health department may not coincide with those of the police department or school system. Finally, survey reports of social indicators (e.g., U.S. Census data) tend to be published at relatively long intervals, while community areas often undergo rapid and significant changes. Overall, social indicators provide only indirect information on the needs in a community.

Field Surveys

Field surveys focus on the general community population and rely on statistical probability sampling procedures. The most important advantage of a field survey is that it can directly access the needs of a representative sample of the community population. In doing so, investigators are able to determine the representativeness of their samples and the generalizability of their findings. In addition, findings derived from large samples are more amenable to tests for validity and reliability and can be tested more appropriately for statistical significance. Moreover, the surveys can be designed to identify the specific needs and service patterns of the general population and of most subpopulations living within a community. For these reasons, surveys provide data that are particularly valuable for planning community health promotion programs (Warheit et al., 1983). Although many researchers agree that scientifically designed and implemented field surveys provide the most valid and worthwhile community needs assessments, the process of conducting an empirical survey may limit the researchers' ability to develop collaborative relations with the participants, to facilitate empowerment, or to understand the more subtle aspects of the community. We will return to these issues later in the chapter.

Key Informants

A fourth method used extensively in conducting community needs assessment consists of relying on the responses of key informants. Elected or appointed political leaders, administrative and program personnel of various service-providing agencies, clergy, teachers, law enforcement personnel, and other community members may provide valuable information regarding the needs/problems of community members. The process of interviewing community members is relatively simple and inexpensive and can provide interesting information, particularly when diverse informants are represented. Of course, the selection of interview subjects may be biased. Groups are usually selected not because they are statistically representative but because of their presumed knowledge about the community. Despite this and other methodological difficulties (see Warheit et al., 1977), the key informant approach enables the interviewer to establish an open dialogue with the participant. Such a rapport ultimately facilitates a deeper understanding of the experiences and needs of the community members and may mobilize action toward community change (Belenky, Clinchy, Goldberger, & Tarule, 1986).

For example, Mies (1983) described an assessment of battered women that included taping interviews and conversations between the participants, listening to them in groups of various sizes, and having all of the participants (researchers and researched) describe their impressions of the assessment process. The aim of this research was not only to assess the needs of these women, but to record a collective experience of women that would lead to strategies for change. By sharing their life histories with each other, it was hoped that these women would be relieved from a sense of personal failure and be motivated to work for change. The project was successful: Not only did the women start finding the determination to change their own situation, but they also began to recognize connections between their lives and the lives of the female researchers. The assessment ultimately resulted in suggestions for changes in the lives of the women. Methods such as this may ultimately convey a more holistic picture of the community assessed.

ISSUES IN COMMUNITY NEEDS ASSESSMENT

Even though many researchers have strong preferences for a particular assessment method, there is no one right way to conduct a community needs assessment. Some researchers may believe that the only way to develop a clear understanding of a social phenomenon is to conduct a true field experiment, whereas others may feel that the richness and complexity of community phenomena may be best understood by careful observation over long periods of time with an open dialogue. Ultimately, however, the choice of methodology depends on the demands of the setting, as well as on (a) the objectives, biases, and values of the person conducting the needs assessment; (b) the desired degree of collaboration; and (c) the choice of the level of analysis appropriate to the community.

Values

Values and objectives can vary widely and greatly influence the specification of needs and communities, the methodology chosen to actually conduct the assessment, and the ways that the results are used and interpreted. By recognizing and articulating our values, we can make decisions in a manner that is more explicit, systematic, and negotiated. For example, the very process of defining a "need" for which to provide resources varies according to our values and objectives. The concept of need from a health promotion and primary prevention standpoint is quite different from that which results from more traditional views (Felner & Aber, 1983). From the traditional perspective, a need may be said to be present when a discrete pathology is identified. Alternatively, community-based psychologists often must identify and define need in such a way that permits its assessment when no problems have become evident in the community.

For example, Rhodes & Jason (1990) report on a community-based substance abuse prevention program for adolescents living in Chicago. The project is being coordinated through a community mental health center, and a central concern raised by the Center's director was about the need for a program for adolescents who weren't substance abusers. From the administrator's perspective, the program seemed a diversion of resources from those adolescents who were really "in need." This concern is warranted; however, waiting for substance abuse to be manifest before attempting to justify service is contrary to the goals of community-based health promotion efforts.

Even when provided with a clear definition of "need," it is often difficult to establish priorities rationally and to determine which needs can be met most effectively by which agencies. The identification of community needs tends to be guided by the values and attitudes of those defining the need. This is because the evaluation and interpretation of needs are influenced by the vested interests of those formulating program goals, the capabilities of the staff, and the availability of appropriate service technology and adequate funding.

The value-based nature of community needs assessment helps to explain the discrepancies that often exist between the actual needs in our society and allocations of resources. Although assessment information may frequently include objective data, planning remains a value-based process. All community programs have a varied group of stakeholders, including elected representatives, program funders, administrators, other community service providers, community residents, and service recipients. These stakeholders may represent diverse vested interests and hold disparate values and expectations. As a result, the task of translating assessment information about community needs into relevant service programs is not a simple, objective process, but rather a complex task that requires decision-making, negotiation, and conciliation.

Because needs assessment strategies are frequently value-based and conducted with a focus on the needs of a particular group within the community, the health needs of other groups often go unnoticed. For example, in the United States, breast cancer is the most common cancer in women, afflicting approximately 1 woman in 10, and is the most frequent cause of cancer death among women (Konner, 1988). Despite the fact that the risk factors have been clearly isolated, research and health promotion programs have been remarkably sparse. In addressing this issue, Konner (1988) points to the value-laden nature of our program priorities:

> *I sometimes wonder what sets our priorities. As with other disenfranchised populations, have breast-cancer patients counted less because they were women?*

Batchelor (1988) articulated similar sentiments with respect to AIDS priorities:

The rampant homophobia within Congress and among many other federal, state, and local government officials will continue to force AIDS prevention programs to be funded out of private donations rather than the public funds that this public health emergency deserves. The limits of science are bounded by the limits of human understanding and empathy. (p. 857)

The relatively slow and inadequate response to the need for AIDS research, treatment, and prevention underscores the fact that our values often point us toward assessing certain issues as opposed to others. As another example of this tendency, significant national attention has focused on childhood abductions, and certainly this is a serious and legitimate problem. The abuse that many more children suffer due to poverty, however, is not given the same type of national attention. Could this, at least in part, be due to the fact that one problem can be seen as caused by identifiable individuals (i.e., the abductor), and thus more straightforward solutions are possible (e.g, find and arrest the perpetrator)? Alternately, the causes of poverty are more systemic and complex, and some solutions might even threaten the lifestyles of mainstream America. In assessing community problems, an evaluator could be influenced by funders or community groups to focus on the problems that have gained more public attention and, as a consequence, other salient issues (e.g., breast cancer, AIDS, poverty) might be ignored. The assessment process might be heavily influenced by the norms and values of our society, and as such, we might ignore important issues.

Despite the inherently value-laden nature of community needs assessment, many researchers assume that it is, for the most part, an objective process. Marti-Costa & Serrano-Garcia (1983) suggest that this "myth of neutrality" distorts the process and is undesirable. Need assessment, they argue, is a political process that can be conceptualized as a tool for organization, mobilization, and consciousness-raising among groups and communities. They state:

Need assessment is an integral part of community development, the process of consciousness-raising. It implies a political commitment which undermines the traditional view of a neutral science and a firm commitment to the exploited, underprivileged, and powerless groups in society.

This viewpoint is compatible with feminist methodology, which tries to take the needs, interests, and experiences of the community into account and aims at improving conditions. This is contrasted with research or assessment "on" the population, which tends to be conducted without careful examination of values or the suitability of the methods (Klein, 1983). A lack of openness and discussion concerning one's values and objectives can create divisions, distrust, and resentment from participants.

Cook and Shadish (1986) suggested that there are three ways to ameliorate social problems: through the incremental modifications in existing social programs, through demonstration program that are ultimately disseminated, and through bringing about changes in social structures and beliefs. The assessment process is influenced by beliefs about how social problems should be addressed. Assessments can be directed toward systemic influences on individuals or on the outcome of these influences. If lack of opportunity is a significant factor in a community, and high rates of crime are a manifestation of this factor, then assessments that fail to account for the opportunity factor are missing a significant component.

Of course, some would contend that there are numerous values (e.g., justice, human rights, equality), some of which might even be contradictory in certain situations, and it is unclear which is needed to advance to a better society (Shadish, 1990). Many program evaluators and community assessors would even take the next step by stating that evaluators need to remain neutral, and in this way they can earn the respect of antagonists in a conflict. There are, no doubt, circumstances where this is the best policy. The stakeholders who fund the assessments, however, might represent the more middle-class segment of the community, and if this is the case, then those with few resources and little power might not have access to the same professional resources as others. In these situations, community assessors could be advocates of those who are unempowered and lacking resources. Assessors working with poverty groups, for example, might focus on additional, more systemic issues, and by collecting information on such factors they bring about an even more balanced representation of the problems facing the community.

Cook and Shadish (1986) cite three theories of evaluation: the *manipulable solutions,* where evaluations focus on discovering solutions and where less importance is accorded with explaining how a phenomena works; the *generalized explanation alternative,* which sees the works as having complex interrelationships where there are multiple causal determinants, and purports that more time needs to be spent on exploratory studies that model theories; and the *stakeholder service* approach, which advocates giving useful information to stakeholders, who will then be in a better position to make majority decisions. Each of these approaches has its benefits and limitations, and perhaps one day we will be able to use multiple models that will even further enrich our assessment strategies.

The efficacy and utilization of the assessment findings will also be enhanced if the evaluator is aware of the values of the agency/manager for whom the assessment is being conducted. The results of even the most carefully conducted needs assessment are infrequently utilized by program managers. This is because needs assessment information is often not relevant to program decisions or carefully explained to program managers. For example, program evaluators and program managers often have different biases toward the form of the information; needs assessors typically present objective or numerical data, while managers tend to distrust such data and often prefer direct, human, subjective, value-weighted input. In order to assure the utilization of needs assessment results, program evaluators should tailor the form of the information to the decision demands and objectives of the agency. Unfortunately, evaluators typically do not really know, understand, or have full access to the program managers' value context. They often are unaware of al the implications of a decision and concentrate instead on their designs, measures, and data analysis. In general, a collaborative approach to needs assessment facilitates an awareness of values and increases the likelihood that the findings will be utilized.

Degree of Collaboration

In collaborative needs assessment, the participants are defined as co-equals in the assessment process and contribute to the decisions about data collection and use (Kelly, 1986). Efforts are made to allow community members to identify their own problems, with professionals acting as resource providers. In this collaborative model, professionals are helping the community members became empowered by providing the resources to enable them to build on their own strengths and develop self-correcting solutions. Preventive interventions engendered by a collaborative, empowering needs assessment process may be more likely to be *truly adopted*, whereas outside solutions that are more or less imposed on a community may be only *manifestly adopted* (Rappaport, Seidman, & Davidson, 1979). For example, in compliance with pressure from parents, a school system may identify needs and manifestly adopt a health promotion curriculum but make no further systemic changes necessary for the program to be fully accepted and disseminated within the setting. In this case, the very nature of the project may be transformed into something that helps the school stay the same and helps local agencies (e.g., treatment programs) maintain the scope of their functions. A program is more likely to be truly adopted into the community when it is consistent with the characteristics, practices, and values of the community.

Kelly (1986) pointed to some of the early antecedents of collaborative research for the field of community assessment. He notes that, in some instances, awareness of the value of collaborative work has come about as a result of marked failures in citizens not responding or not having opportunities to influence planned interventions or assessment procedures. Community members tend to be skeptical of assessment procedures, fearing that the researcher might exploit them and their histories. For example, we recently interviewed a group of teachers who reported that they were deliberately withholding important information from the university-based assessor in an effort to undermine the effort. The reason for these actions was clear: They did not feel respected or understood by the assessor and suspected that their contributions would ultimately benefit her career. Had the researcher taken the time to establish rapport, find meaningful, collaborative roles for the participants, and understand their values and needs vis-à-vis the assessment, this difficult situation might have been avoided.

Collaborative research also details a recognition that the "truth" of a person or community cannot be asked for, is not static, but grows and develops over time (Mies, 1983). Because the needs of an individual are relative, they should be recorded in an interactive rather than linear way. By combining our empirical procedures with an openness to subjective experience and interactions over time, we may produce findings that better encompass the complexity of a community (Klein, 1983).

Level of Analysis

Another subtle but critical issue to consider when conducting needs assessment involves the unit of analysis appropriate to the phenomena of interest. Community processes may be studied at several different levels, and decisions about this issue will have an important influence on a number of other assessment decisions to be made. For example, in assessing the need for health promotion services within several school districts, the researcher could compare the incidence of health disorder among individual students, whole classes, schools, or even school districts. Communities can be thought of as consisting of several levels of social organization, including individuals, groups, organizations, and communities. Community and social phenomena, such as family and school behaviors, should be studied from the perspective of one or several of these levels of analysis. Psychologists tend to concern themselves with understanding behavior and assessing needs at only two levels of analysis—the individual and the group levels—and focus less on the organizational and community levels. This has overshadowed the notable ways that various and multiple levels of social organization subtly influence social behaviors and communities (Shinn, in press).

Consider again the issue of substance use among adolescents. Researchers who focus exclusively on individual characteristics (e.g., resistance to peer pressure, assertiveness, self-esteem) may fail to take into account crucial variables that operate at other levels of analysis, such as the peer or family group, community tolerance for usage, opportunities for alternative activities, or the amount and quality of resources possessed by a youth's school and community (Rhodes & Jason, 1988).

A failure to appreciate the ecological context produces assessment results that are less comprehensive and useful. Such an approach constricts our understanding of problem behavior. For example, although drug dealing and gang activity are unequivocally delinquent behaviors, they offer extremely powerful contingencies (e.g., status, money, independence, mobility) to youth residing in impoverished neighborhoods. An individual assessment might also miss the fact that many children need to walk to school through different territories controlled by gangs. If they join a gang, they decrease the probability of being picked on or beaten up (Thompson & Jason, 1988). Similarly, although teen pregnancy can be seen as quite dysfunctional and antithetical to education and career, it too provides many of the same contingencies for young women that drug dealing and gang activity provide for young men (e.g., status, a visible product, social and financial support). Additionally, both behaviors provide a developmental marker into adulthood, much the same as college or the military service do for middle-class youth. When we expand our conceptual framework and consider the contingencies and norms of the settings, behaviors that once appeared pathogenic often appear quite functional. To the extent that one assesses individual factors in understanding a child's ability to resist joining a gang or engaging in unprotected sexuality, many influential factors are ignored and ultimately the solutions fall short.

Overall, our assessment of communities can be enhanced considerably by taking into account the complex transactions among variables operating at multiple levels of analysis. When the needs of individuals are presented with regard to the social, economic, environmental, or political context, decision-makers are in a better position to move beyond individually centered solutions.

FUTURE DIRECTIONS

In the previous sections, we have argued that effective community needs assessment requires the use of careful methodology, a collaborative framework, and concepts and approaches that illuminate subjective experiences and transactions between individuals and social settings. Although these approaches are conceptually appealing, the movement of this position into the everyday concerns of needs assessment can be difficult. This is because an ecological and collaborative framework means interactions and complexity and points us toward analysis and intervention in larger-scale systems. To the extent that solutions challenge the distribution of resources and call for structural changes in social and economic systems, they will likely be resisted. Nonetheless, assessment at various levels can broaden our understanding of needs and ultimately assist in the generation of optimal solutions and services.

A second major goal of this chapter has been to challenge the assumptions and techniques that underlie traditional assessment. More specifically, we are calling into question the traditional model of assessment, which establishes "truth" by objective, dispassionate, and presumably value-free methods. We have suggested that our current assessment methods, which rely largely on the collecting, coding, and statistical analysis of data, may tell us very little about a community. From our perspective, the most holistic understanding and assessment of needs will probably emerge through empathic and honest dialogue with various community members. This point was exemplified during an assessment conducted recently at a reform school outside of a major metropolitan area. Adolescents charged with drug dealing, usage, or related delinquent behaviors are typically sent to this boarding school for a period of 12 months. All of our assessment interviews were conducted with strict confidentiality, and efforts were made to impart an atmosphere of trust and openness. Our first inquiries as to the extent of drug use on campus were made to senior staff, many of whom were disconnected from (and disliked by) the teaching staff and students. The senior staff informed us that drug use was strictly prohibited on school grounds, that "strip searches" were conducted regularly, and that there was little or no use among the students. Our next set of inquiries were made to the teaching staff, whose responses ranged from describing rampant drug use to reporting virtually no use. Finally, a group of students described to us an extensive drug-dealing network within the dormitories that was patterned after their urban neighborhoods. This scenario underscores the importance of moving beyond traditional forms of knowledge attainment and needs assessment. The reports and discrepancies signify both the need for more appropriate services and the lack of communication and collaboration among staff and students.

Belenky and others (1986) distinguished two forms of procedural knowledge, understanding versus knowledge. Understanding involves intimacy and equality between the assessor and the object, while knowledge implies separation from the object and mastery over it. Understanding is the basis for *connected knowing* and entails acceptance and an attempt to enter the other person's frame of mind to discover the premises for the other's point of view. Feminist theorists have described this process as the *context of discovery* (Harding & O'Barr, 1987; Hare-Mustin & Maracek, 1988), emphasizing dialogue and listening as the key components of connected knowing.

Given social scientists' traditional reliance on self-reports and nonintrusive measures, it could be argued that a methodology that is based on collaboration and dialogue could reduce objectivity. Such methodology, however, when conducted in a clear and consistent manner, can provide rich and objective data. One of the meanings of objectivity is that people do not project their own values and agendas onto the external object. Traditionally, assessors have avoided this by suppressing the self, taking as impersonal a stance as possible toward the object. Alternatively, connected knowing is built on the conviction that the most trustworthy knowledge comes from personal experience. Connected knowers develop strategies to access others' knowledge, and central to these procedures is the capacity for empathy. Insofar as is possible, assessors should strive to be connected rather than separate, seeing the community not in the assessors' terms but in the members' terms. This will permit the researcher to constantly compare the assessment work with his or her own experiences and to share it with the researched, who then add their opinions to the assessment, which in turn might change it.

Ecologically sensitive community needs assessments may emerge through the integration of traditional methodology with an openness to intuition and feelings. In combination with our intellectual capacities for analyzing and interpreting our observations, this open acknowledgement of the interactions of facts and feelings might produce an assessment that encompasses the complexity of community.

REFERENCES

Baker, M. (1974). *The design of human service systems.* Wellesley, MA: The Human Ecology Institute.

Batchelor, W. F. (1988). AIDS 1988: The science and the limits of science. *American Psychologist, 43,* 853–858.

Belenky, M. F., Clinchy, B. M., Goldberger, N. R., & Tarule, J. M. (1986). *Women's ways of knowing: The development of self, voice, and mind.* New York: Basic Books.

Cook, T. D., & Shadish, W. R. (1986). Program evaluation: The worldly science. In M. R. Rosenzweig & L. W. Porter (Eds.), *Annual review of psychology.* Palo Alto: Annual Reviews, Inc.

Cox, G. B., Carmichael, S. J., & Dightman, C. R. (1979). The optional treatment approach to needs assessment. *Evaluation and Program Planning, 2,* 269–275.

Felner, R. D., & Aber, M. S. (1983). Primary prevention for children: A framework for the assessment of need. *Prevention in Human Services, 2*(4), 9–33.

Felner, R. D., & Felner, T. Y. (in press). Primary prevention programs in the educational context: A transactional framework and analysis. In L. Bond & B. Compas (Eds.), *Primary prevention in the schools.* Beverly Hills: Sage Publications.

Harding, S., & O'Barr, J. F. (1987). *Sex and scientific inquiry.* Chicago: The University of Chicago Press.

Hare-Mustin, R. T., & Marecek, J. (1988). The meaning of difference: Gender, theory, postmodernism, and psychology. *American Psychologist, 43*(6), 455–465.

Jason, L. A., & Liotta, R. F. (1982). Assessing community responsiveness in a metropolitan area. *Evaluation Review, 6*(5), 703–712.

Kelly, J. G. (1986). Context and process: An ecological view of the interdependence of practice and research. *American Journal of Community Psychology, 14,* 581–589.

Klein, R. D. (1983). How to do what we want to do: Thoughts about feminist methodology. In G. Bowles & R. Klein (Eds.), *Theories of women's studies.* Boston: Routledge & Kegan Paul.

Konner, M. (1988, November 20). Civilization's cancer. *New York Times Magazine,* pp. 66–67.

Marti-Costa, S., & Serrano-Garcia, I. (1983). Needs assessment and community development: An ideological perspective. *Prevention in Human Services, 2*(4), 9–33.

Mies, M. (1983). Towards a methodology for feminist research. In G. Bowles & R. Klein (Eds.), *Theories of women's studies.* Boston: Routledge & Kegan Paul.

Rappaport, J., Seidman, E., & Davidson, W. (1979). Demonstration research and manifestation versus true adoption: The natural history of a research project to divert adolescents from the legal system. In R. F. Munoz, L. Snow, & J. Kelly (Eds.), *Social and psychological research in community settings.* San Francisco: Jossey Bass.

Rhodes, J. E., & Jason, L. A. (1988). *Preventing substance abuse among children and adolescents.* New York: Pergamon.

Rhodes, J. E., & Jason, L. A. (in press). A social stress model of substance abuse. *Journal of Consulting and Clinical Psychology.*

Shadish, W. R. (1990). Criteria for excellence in community research. In P. Tolan, C. Keys, F. Chertok, & L. A. Jason (Eds.), *Researching community psychology.* Washington, DC: American Psychological Association.

Shinn, M. B. (in press). Mixing and matching levels of analysis. In P. Tulan, L. A. Jason, et al. (Eds.), *Researching community psychology: Integrating theories and methodologies.* Washington, DC: American Psychological Association.

Siegel, C., Attkisson, C. C., & Carson, L. G. (1978). Evaluation of human service programs. In C. C. Attkisson, W. A. Hargreaves, M. J. Horowitz, & J. E. Sorensen (Eds.), *Evaluation of human service programs* (pp. 215–251). New York: Academic Press.

Siegel, L. M., Attkisson, C. C., & Cohn, A. H. (1977). Mental health needs assessment: Strategies and techniques. In W. A. Hargreaves, C. C. Attkisson, & J. E. Sorensen (Eds.), *Resource materials for community mental health program evaluation* (2nd ed.) (DHEW Publication NO. ADM 77-328). Washington, DC: U.S. Government Printing Office.

Thompson, D. W., & Jason, L. A. (1988). Street gangs and preventive interventions. *Criminal Justice and Behavior, 15*(3), 323–333.

Warheit, G., Bell, R., & Schwab, J. (1977). *Needs assessment approaches: Concepts and methods* (DHEW Publication No. ADM 77-472). Washington, DC: U.S. Government Printing Office.

Warheit, G. J., Vega, W. A., & Buhl-Auth, J. (1983). Mental health needs assessment approaches: A case for applied epidemiology. *Prevention in Human Services, 2*(4), 9–33.

Zautra, A., & Simons, L. S. (1978). An assessment of a community's mental health needs. *American Journal of Community Psychology, 6,* 351–362.

Index

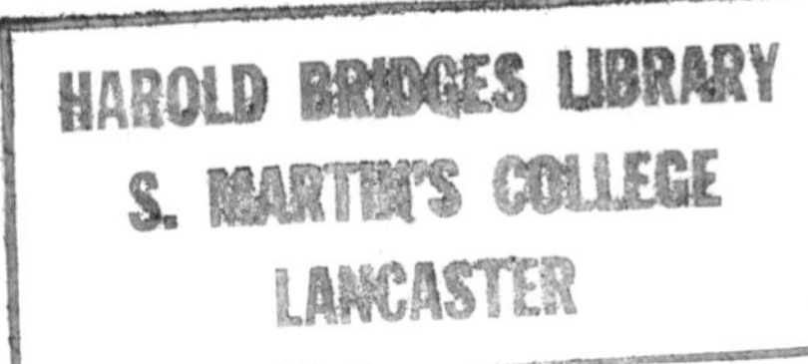